THE BLACK DEATH

THE
BLACK DEATH
A Turning Point in History?

Edited by **WILLIAM M. BOWSKY**
University of California, Davis

ROBERT E. KRIEGER PUBLISHING COMPANY
MALABAR, FLORIDA

Cover illustration: Victims of the Black Death being buried in mass graves, Tournai, Belgium, 1349. From a contemporary manuscript. *(The Granger Collection)*

Original Edition 1971
Reprint 1978

Printed and Published by
ROBERT E. KRIEGER PUBLISHING COMPANY, INC.
KRIEGER DRIVE
MALABAR, FL 32950

Copyright © 1971 by
HOLT, RINEHART & WINSTON
Reprinted by Arrangement

Printed in the United States of America

Library of Congress Cataloging in Publication Data

Bowsky, William M   comp.
  The Black Death.

  Reprint of the ed. published by Holt, Rinehart and Winston, New York, in series: European problem studies.
  Bibliography: p.
  1. Black death—Addresses, essays, lectures.
  2. Diseases and history—Addresses, essays, lectures.
I. Title.
[RC172.B67   1978]   940.1-7   77-21196
ISBN 0-88275-636-2

10 9 8 7 6 5 4

CONTENTS

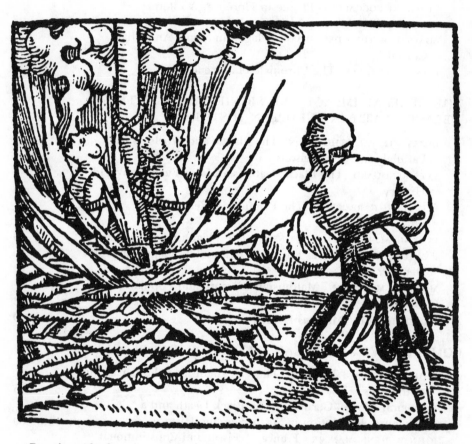

Burning of plague spreaders. From Sebastian Münster, *Cosmographia Universalis. (Bettmann Archive)*

INTRODUCTION

One of our most pressing concerns today is that mankind may unleash upon itself the holocaust of a nuclear war whose fire storm, fallout, and radiation would dwarf the horrors of the atomic destruction of Hiroshima and Nagasaki in 1945. Six centuries ago European civilization experienced a frighteningly analogous disaster: at least one out of four men, women, and children, more than twenty million in all, died terribly—victims of what came to be called the Black Death. The toll was at least double the number of those who perished in western Europe during World War II.

The evil that confronted our late medieval forebears was even worse in some ways than that which we ourselves contemplate. We can anticipate the catastrophe intellectually, if not emotionally, and, perhaps more important, we act as though we believe that our own actions, if wisely chosen, can avert it. Men of the four-teenth century were ignorant of the affliction that assailed them. They lacked the knowledge with which to respond or save themselves. And when it early ap-peared that prayers and pious intercession were of no avail, fear could lead to a broad if not always attractive range of manifestations of intense religiosity and emotion.

The horror known as the Black Death of 1348 resulted from a complex com-bination of events whose nature has become known only in recent years. The plague bacillus, *Pasturella pestis,* is common among certain rodents and ordi-narily causes them only mild infection and few fatalities. But when infected ro-dents live in close proximity to humans and are heavily infested with a particular type of flea *(Xenopsylla cheopis),* the situation changes radically. This flea is so constructed that its sucking mechanism is easily blocked when it is laden with plague bacilli. That valvular obstruction prevents the flea from feeding by suck-ing in blood. Instead it ejects deadly plague bacilli as it repeatedly punctures its victim in vain attempts to feed.

All too common in the mid-fourteenth century was the black rat *(Rattus rattus),* which is accustomed to live close to men and whose fleas are among those that will attack humans most readily.[1] From those fleas there first spread the

---

[1] The displacement of the black rat by the more rural and more ferocious brown rat *(R. norvegicus)* in the eighteenth century helps to account for the termination of a long series of plague epidemics in western Europe.

1

bubonic plague, so called from the buboes, or swellings, that appear in the areas of the victim's lymph glands. Some sufferers of bubonic plague contracted pneumonia, and from it the far more deadly pneumonic plague. This extremely infectious airborne disease is almost always fatal—ordinarily within only four days. (As men do not develop immunity to pneumonic plague, it apparently died out only when a sufficient number of victims became infected so rapidly and heavily that they never lived long enough to reach the coughing stage.) Nor were men spared septicemic plague, which occurs only in the most severe outbreaks. With this type of plague the sufferer's bloodstream became infected so heavily that there was no time for buboes to appear; victims often died within a few hours. All three varieties of plague cursed Europe from late 1347 through 1350.

This catastrophe burned itself indelibly into the minds of contemporaries, and survivors wrote of it vividly and in minute detail, as is seen from the readings in the first section. The most famous account was composed during the years immediately following the disaster of 1348. It is contained in the introduction to the *Decameron,* the vernacular prose masterpiece of the Florentine humanist Giovanni Boccaccio. Its powerful descriptions of the epidemic's course and of its effects in the Florentine city and countryside are strikingly dramatic. It is instructive to compare this polished literary description with that of a chronicler, Agnolo di Tura del Grasso ("the Fat"), from the city of Siena, less than forty miles south of Florence. Reporting on the plague was not restricted to Italians or to laymen. A most interesting account is that of a French Carmelite friar, Jean de Venette. In comparing his treatment of the plague with those of Boccaccio and Agnolo it is worth sorting out the similarities and the differences in emphasis, nuance, description, and values. Which variations may be ascribed to contrasts between clerics and laymen, Italians (or Tuscans!) and northern Europeans, which to personal characteristics, and which indeed may result from the plague having taken a diverse course or suscitated quite varied responses in the different parts of Europe? (And it would be a mistake simply to discard these medieval eyewitness accounts when they do not seem to accord with more recent "scientific" interpretations.)

Shared by all survivors was a stunned horror at the magnitude of the disaster. Nor is this surprising since even low modern estimates reckon the loss of life in the first epidemic, of 1348, to have been no less than one-fourth of the population of Europe. This alone would lead one to expect that its effects were enormous. Indeed many opponents of this view seem essentially to be trying to explain away connections between the plague and various changes that occurred in postplague Europe, and to argue that such connections do not in fact exist but merely result from the fallacy of *post hoc* reasoning—the assumption that because one thing follows another there is a causal relationship between them.

To many modern writers it seems more reasonable to hold the opposite view, and, in fact, to regard the Black Death of the mid-fourteenth century as one of the epoch-making events in history and a major factor in bringing about significant historical change. Specifically, it has been linked to the end of a medieval civilization and the beginning of the modern world. Cardinal Francis Aidan Gasquet put the case clearly in 1893 in *The Great Pestilence*. Among its consequences in England he cites "the overthrow of the mediaeval system of serfdom," the change from a French to an English literary culture, a "great dearth of [secular] clergy," and a loss of zeal among the monastic clergy of postplague decades. He quotes approvingly "that the steady progress of the twelfth and thirteenth centuries was suddenly checked in the fourteenth . . . the Black Death swept off half the population and the whole social structure was disorganized." "The plague," wrote Gasquet, "simply shattered [existing institutions]." Writing large he saw the Black Death as the watershed between a Middle Ages marked by hope and optimism and the "practical pessimism" that he found too common in modern times.

This position was not abandoned in the twentieth century. The late George G. Coulton, a prolific and polemical medieval historian, inclined toward it in his short book *The Black Death* (1929). He wrote that "this catastrophe . . . contributed to hasten that impulse of independent research which we call the Renaissance, and that religious revolution, closely akin to it which we call the Reformation. . . . It will probably be more and more recognized that the Black Death does, in fact, begin a new epoch in medieval society. . . . the plague shook, even shattered, many things which were already decaying or unstable; while . . . institutions founded solidly on deep human needs and movements inspired by elementary natural impulses, after the first shock, grew onwards . . . at an increasing rate."

In reading the following selections the student might weigh the extent to which a single historical phenomenon, in this case the plague, appears to have either marked or brought about significant turning points in various areas of human endeavor and in the value systems commonly shared by European men. Where did the Black Death serve as a catalyst for changes that had already begun? Where did it apparently have no lasting effects? Consider carefully, too, the presumptions brought to each argument, the types of questions posed, and the nature of the evidence adduced by the scholars who address themselves to the problem of the Black Death.

In the second section of this book we examine a few of the more important writings on the general impact and significance of the Black Death in European history.

The slaughter and upheaval of World War I horrified men and brought some historians to think back to other great disasters of Western history. The medievalist James Westfall Thompson puts forth a series of analogies and parallels between the "Great War" of his own generation and the Black Death. Some readers may be surprised at the apparent modernity of certain of his comparisons or at his use of psychology. All should try to ascertain the degree, if any, to which the comparison seems forced or the evidence tailored to fit a Procrustean bed. Emphasis upon the impact of the plague is not confined to those shaken by World War I. As recently as 1969 the economic historian Harry A. Miskimin wrote that "The most far-reaching event of the later Middle Ages was beyond doubt the plague of 1348–49, reinforced in its effects by its subsequent recurrences. . . . "[2]

Recent decades have seen a spate of research related to the plague, but far from a unanimity of opinion, as scholars posed new and more varied questions. In surveying the plague from numerous vantage points and considering its total impact on Europe, Yves Renouard comes to the conclusion that it was indeed a major event in world history. Élisabeth Carpentier argues that the plague's impact can be seen properly only by viewing the disaster as a recurrent phenomenon, to be seen as a totality, and not by confining our attention to the first great epidemic of the mid-fourteenth century.

The Russian scholar Evgenii Alekseevich Kosminskii takes an entirely different tack in a lucid illustration of the application of Marxist theory to a major historical problem: he considers the plague in relation to the broad question of the economic development of western Europe during the fourteenth and fifteenth centuries. Kosminskii directly attacks the theory held by a majority of Western historians that this was a period of economic depression. In the course of his provocative analysis he plays down the role of the plague as an important causative factor in economic history.

Raymond Delatouche also deemphasizes the significance of the Black Death, but for far different reasons. Attacking the Malthusian argument that a demographic crisis first occurred prior to the plague because the population had outstripped the ability of agriculture to support it, he holds that agricultural production could have been increased sufficiently to maintain a growing population. Delatouche contends that the crisis of European civilization occurred more than a half century before the Black Death, and was essentially a crisis of morale and morality. The Black Death simply furthered the decline. Much of his argumentation deals with France, and the student is invited to compare it with the discussion of the plague in that country by other authors in this book, including Jean de Venette, and to determine how much France and the impact of the plague there were typical of Europe.

The Malthusian argument and the case for an economic depression that started well before the arrival of the plague is best made by Michael M. Postan. He holds that increasing population had led men to cultivate marginal lands, lands whose fertility soon was exhausted and their yield diminished. Conceding that the fourteenth-century epidemics "decimated population," Postan suggests

---

[2] Harry A. Miskimin, *The Economy of Early Renaissance Europe, 1300–1460* (New York: Prentice-Hall, Inc., 1969), p. 134.

that "recovery was slow and fitful" because "population and production in any case were moving downwards."

While agreeing that the Tuscan population had been declining for at least a half century before the Black Death, David Herlihy completely rejects a Malthusian explanation, and he poses a fascinating alternative in the course of a provocative study of the Tuscan town of Pistoia. He suggests that "Although natural disasters clearly played a role of major importance in Pistoia's demographic history, their impact was apparently aggravated, and recovery from them delayed, by a low and unresponsive birth rate." The reader will want to examine carefully how historians who agree upon certain specific data or even long-term trends arrive at differing, even diametrically opposed interpretations.

The third section of readings allows us to test some of the broad generalizations presented earlier against the results of specific case studies for more limited regions. Were the plague's effects everywhere the same and of equal intensity? If there was variety, what caused it? Do scholars viewing the same localities reach harmonious or contrasting conclusions—and to what extent does this depend upon the questions they pose or the facets of life upon which they concentrate?

Examining the plague in Germany, Philip Ziegler sees its peculiar manifestations there in religious and psychological excesses that gave rise to the masochism of self-flagellation and to bestial persecution of the Jews. One might ask why the virulence of these phenomena was particularly great in Germany. Friedrich Lütge has a different vantage point, and claims that in Germany the plague unleashed a structural revolution in socioeconomic history. And if one can agree with John B. Henneman, Jr., its impact was no less in France—if we focus upon constitutional and fiscal issues. Yet it is intriguing to compare these studies and hypotheses with Charles Verlinden's analysis of the situation in Spain. He concludes that in Spain the plague had no fundamental consequence, a "conclusion" that he believes "is valid for all of Europe."

Much research related to the Black Death has concentrated upon England because of the richness of its archival sources. The treatment by George A. Holmes is far more modern and sophisticated than that of Cardinal Gasquet. For this reason it is especially interesting to see that it follows in the same tradition of interpretation. Holmes sees the Black Death as one of the few truly decisive turning points in English history, and argues his case from cultural as well as social and economic developments. He accepts, however, the argumentation of Postan that preplague England already was overpopulated, with land scarce, and wages low. These contentions are challenged by Josiah C. Russell in a selection from a scholarly article that permits the reader to examine and evaluate some of the fascinating techniques developed for the study of medieval demography as used by a pioneer and outstanding expert in this rapidly developing discipline.

Italy was the Western land first struck by the Black Death, and apparently one of those that suffered the most. A particularly challenging examination of the plague in Italy is a detailed and technical analysis by the art historian Millard Meiss. From his *Painting in Florence and Siena after the Black Death* (1959) there emerges the theme that the crises of the 1340s, and the plague above all, evoked both spiritual and artistic responses. Meiss finds that postplague art, with its emphasis on the remoteness and majesty of divinity, resembles more closely the art of the thirteenth century than the more optimistic art of the half century that preceded the epidemic.

In the next selection Élisabeth Carpentier moves from a general considera-tion of the Black Death to its impact upon the central Italian hill town of Orvieto, about halfway between Florence and Rome. Most striking is the contrast between her assessment of the plague's political, social, and economic effects on the one hand, and its personal and psychological impact on the other. An analogous study of the neighboring hill town of Siena by William M. Bowsky yields some-what different results. Is this because of differences in the questions posed by or the source materials available to each scholar, or due more to actual differ-ences in plague impact and town response—and why, indeed, should these have differed?

Abraham L. Udovitch takes us across the Mediterranean into Egypt. He argues that a demographic crisis brought on by the Black Death was a major factor in the economic decline of that land. His findings for Muslim Egypt can be compared fruitfully with what we have learned of the role of the plague in Christian Europe.

Analyses of the plague, its impact and significance, have become more re-fined and nuanced in recent decades. They involve and interrelate an increasing number of disciplines, from demography to art history and psychology. Care is being taken to distinguish the initial from the cumulative impact of the mor-tality and its short- and long-term results. Historians are examining the diversity of its effects on differing regions and groups in society. This precision has not been at the expense of missing the forest for the trees and neglecting broad issues of historical change. Scholars continue to probe the relationship of the Black Death to long-term trends in economic history, to the decline of medieval civili-zation, and to the coming of the Renaissance, the Reformation, and our own modern world in a study of what hopefully will continue to rank as the greatest demographic catastrophe to befall Western civilization.

In the reprinted selections footnotes appearing in the original sources have in general been omitted unless they contribute to the argument or better understanding of the selection.

The humanist and classicist GIOVANNI BOCCACCIO (1313–1375), son of a Florentine merchant, was trained in canon law. He became an avid collector of classical manuscripts and a versatile author in both poetry and prose. Boccaccio is best known for his novel the *Decameron,* a collection of tales that were supposedly told by ten young men and women who fled to the countryside to avoid the plague of 1348 and passed the time telling stories. The following passage is the most famous literary description of the Black Death.*

Giovanni Boccaccio

Plague in Florence:
A Literary Description

I say, then, that the years of the era of the fruitful Incarnation of the Son of God had attained to the number of one thousand three hundred and forty-eight, when into the notable city of Florence, fair over every other of Italy, there came the death-dealing pestilence, which, through the operation of the heavenly bodies or of our own iniquitous dealings, being sent down upon mankind for our correction by the just wrath of God, had some years before appeared in the parts of the East, and after having bereft these latter of an innumerable number of inhabitants, extending without cease from one place to another, had now unhappily spread towards the West. And thereagainst no wisdom availing nor human foresight (whereby the city was purged of many impurities by officers deputed to that end and it was forbidden unto any sick person to enter therein and many were the counsels given for the preservation of health) nor yet humble supplications, not once but many times both in ordered processions and in other ways made unto God by devout persons—about the coming in of the Spring of the aforesaid year, it began in a horrible and miraculous way to show forth its dolorous effects. Yet not as it had done in the East, where, if any bled at the nose, it was a manifest sign of inevitable death; nay, but in men and women alike there appeared at the beginning of the malady, certain swellings, either on the groin or under the armpits, whereof some waxed of the

*Adapted from *Stories of Boccaccio (The Decameron),* translated by John Payne (London, n.d.), pp. 1–8.

bigness of a common apple, others like unto an egg, some more and some less, and these the vulgar named plague-boils. From these two parts the aforesaid death-bearing plague-boils proceeded, in brief space, to appear and come indifferently in every part of the body; wherefrom, after awhile, the fashion of the contagion began to change into black or livid blotches, which showed themselves in many first on the arms and about the thighs and after spread to every other part of the person, in some large and sparse and in others small and thick-sown; and like as the plague-boils had been first (and yet were) a very certain token of coming death, even so were these for every one to whom they came.

To the cure of these maladies neither counsel of physician nor virtue of any medicine appeared to avail or profit aught; on the contrary—whether it was that the nature of the infection suffered it not or that the ignorance of the physicians . . . availed not to know whence it arose and consequently took not due measures thereagainst—not only did few recover thereof, but well nigh all died within the third day from the appearance of the aforesaid signs, this one sooner and that later, and for the most part without fever or other accident. And this pestilence was the more virulent because by communication with those who were sick thereof, it got hold upon the sound, as fire upon things dry or greasy, when they are brought very near thereunto. Nay, the harm was yet greater; for that not only did conversation and consorting with the sick give infection to the sound or cause of common death, but the mere touching of the clothes or of whatsoever other thing had been touched or used by the sick appeared of itself to communicate the malady to the toucher. A marvellous thing to hear is that which I have to tell and one which, had it not been seen of many men's eyes and of mine own, I had scarce dared credit, much less set down in writing, though I had heard it from one worthy of belief. I say, then, that of such efficience was the nature of the pestilence in question in communicating itself from one to another, that, not only did it pass from man to man, but this, which is much more, it many times visibly did; to wit, a thing which had pertained to a man sick or dead of the aforesaid sickness, being touched by an animal foreign to the human species, not only infected this latter with the plague; but in a very brief space of time killed it. Of this mine own eyes . . . had one day, among others, experience, to wit, that the rags of a poor man, who had died of the plague, being cast out into the public way, two hogs came up to them and having first, after their wont, rooted amain among them with their snouts, took them in their mouths and tossed them about their jaws; then, in a little while, after turning round and round, they both, as if they had taken poison, fell down dead upon the rags with which they had in an ill hour intermeddled.

From these things and many others like unto them or yet stranger divers fears and conceits were begotten in those who abode alive, which well nigh all tended to a very barbarous conclusion, namely, to shun and flee from the sick and all that pertained to them, and thus doing, each thought to secure immunity for himself. Some there were who conceived that to live moderately and keep one's self from all excess was the best defence against such a danger; wherefore, making up their company, they lived removed from every other and shut themselves up in those houses where none had been sick and where living was best; and there, using very temperately of the most delicate viands and the finest wines and eschewing all incontinence, they abode with music and such other diversions as they might have, never suffering themselves to speak with any nor choosing to hear any news from without of death or sick folk. Others, inclining to the contrary opinion, maintained that to carouse and make merry and go about singing and frolicking and satisfy the appetite in everything possible and laugh and scoff at whatsoever befell was a very certain remedy for such an ill. That which they said they put in practice as best they might, going about day and night, now to this tavern, now to that, drinking without stint or measure; and on this wise they did yet more freely in other folk's houses, if they just scented there anything that pleased or tempted them, as they might lightly do, for every one—as if he were to live no longer—had abandoned all care of his possessions, as of himself, wherefore the most part of the houses were become common good and strangers used them, when they happened upon them, as the very owner might have done; and with all this bestial preoccupation, they still shunned the sick to the best of their power.

In this sore affliction and misery of our city, the reverend authority of the laws, both human and divine, was all in a manner dissolved and fallen into decay, for lack of the ministers and executors thereof, who, like other men, were all either dead or sick or else left so destitute of followers that they were unable to exercise any office, wherefore every one had license to do whatsoever pleased him. Many others held a middle course between the two aforesaid, not straitening themselves so exactly in the matter of diet as the first, neither allowing themselves such license in drinking and other debauchery as the second, but using things in sufficiency, according to their appetites; nor did they seclude themselves, but went about, carrying in their hands, some flowers, some odoriferous herbs and other some divers kinds of spices, which they set often to their noses, accounting it an excellent thing to fortify the brain with such odors, more by token that the air seemed all heavy and attainted with the stench of the dead bodies and that of the sick and of the remedies used.

Some were of a more barbarous, though, perhaps, a surer way of thinking, avouching that there was no remedy against pestilence better than—no, nor any so good as—to flee before them; wherefore, moved by this reasoning and recking of nought but themselves, very many, both men and women, abandoned their own city, their own houses and homes, their kinsfolk and possessions, and sought the country seats of others, or, at the least, their own, as if the wrath of God, being moved to punish the iniquity of mankind, would not proceed to do so wheresoever they might be, but would content itself with afflicting those only who were found within the walls of their city, or as if they were persuaded that no person was to remain therein and that its last hour was come. And albeit these, who opined thus variously, died not all, yet neither did they all escape; nay, many of each way of thinking and in every place sickened of the plague and languished on all sides, well nigh abandoned, having themselves, what while they were whole, set the example to those who abode in health.

Indeed, leaving be that townsman avoided townsman and that well nigh no neighbor took thought unto other and that kinsfolk seldom or never visited one another and held no converse together save from afar, this tribulation had stricken such terror to the hearts of all, men and women alike, that brother forsook brother, uncle nephew and sister brother and oftentimes wife husband; nay (what is yet more extraordinary and well nigh incredible) fathers and mothers refused to visit or tend their very children, as though they had not been theirs. By reason whereof there remained unto those (and the number of them, both males and females, was incalculable) who fell sick, none other succor than that which they owed either to the charity of friends (and of these there were few) or the greed of servants, who tended them, allured by high and extravagant wage; albeit, for all this, these latter were not grown many, and those men and women of mean understanding and for the most part unused to such offices, who served for well nigh nought but to reach things called for by the sick or to note when they died; and in the doing of these services many of them perished with their gain.

Of this abandonment of the sick by neighbors, kinsfolk and friends and of the scarcity of servants arose an usage before well nigh unheard, to wit, that no woman, how fair or lovesome or well-born soever she might be, once fallen sick, recked aught of having a man to tend her, whatever he might be, or young or old, and without any shame discovered to him every part of her body, no otherwise than she would have done to a woman, so but the necessity of her sickness required it; the which belike, in those who recovered, was the occasion of lesser modesty in time to come. Moreover, there ensued of this abandonment the death of many who peradventure, had they been succored, would have escaped alive; wherefore, as

well for the lack of the opportune services which the sick availed not to have as for the virulence of the plague, such was the multitude of those who died in the city by day and by night that it was an astonishment to hear tell thereof, much more to see it; and thence, as it were of necessity, there sprang up among those who abode alive things contrary to the pristine manners of the townsfolk.

It was then (even as we yet see it used) a custom that the kinswomen and she-neighbors of the dead should assemble in his house and there condole with those who more nearly pertained unto him, whilst his neighbors and many other citizens gathered with his next of kin before his house, whither, according to the dead man's quality, came the clergy, and he with funeral pomp of chants and candles was borne on the shoulders of his peers to the church chosen by himself before his death; which usages, after the virulence of the plague began to increase, were either altogether or for the most part laid aside, and other and strange customs sprang up in their stead. For that, not only did folk die without having a multitude of women about them, but many there were who departed this life without witness and few indeed were they to whom the pious plaints and bitter tears of their kinsfolk were vouchsafed; nay, in lieu of these things there obtained, for the most part, laughter and jests and gibes and feasting and merrymaking in company; which usance women, laying aside womanly pitifulness, had right well learned for their own safety.

Few, again, were they whose bodies were accompanied to the church by more than half a score or a dozen of their neighbors, and of these no worshipful and illustrious citizens, but a sort of blood-suckers, sprung from the dregs of the people, who styled themselves *pickmen* and did such offices for hire, shouldered the bier and bore it with hurried steps, not to that church which the dead man had chosen before his death, but most times to the nearest, behind five or six priests, with little light and sometimes none at all, which latter, with the aid of the said pickmen, thrust him into whatever grave they first found unoccupied, without troubling themselves with too long or too formal a service.

The condition of the common people (and belike, in great part, of the middle class also) was yet more pitiable to behold, for these, for the most part retained by hope or poverty in their houses and abiding in their own quarters, sickened by the thousand daily and being altogether untended and unsuccored died well nigh all without recourse. Many breathed their last in the open street, whilst other many, for all they died in their houses, made it known to the neighbors that they were dead rather by the stench of their rotting bodies than otherwise; and the whole city was full of these and others who died all about. For the most part one same usance was observed by the neighbors, moved more by fear lest the corruption of the dead bodies should imperil themselves than by any charity they had for the departed; to wit, that either with their own hands or with the aid of certain bearers, when they might have any, they brought the bodies of those who had died forth of their houses and laid them before their doors, where especially in the morning, those who went about might see corpses without number; then they fetched biers and some, in default thereof, they laid upon some board or other. Nor was it only one bier that carried two or three corpses, nor did this happen but once; nay, many might have been counted which contained husband and wife, two or three brothers, father and son or the like. And an infinite number of times it befell that, two priests going with one cross for some one, three or four biers, borne by bearers, ranged themselves behind the latter, and whereas the priests thought to have but one dead man to bury, they had six or eight, and sometimes more. Nor therefore were the dead honored with any tears or candles or funeral train; nay, the thing was come to such a pass that folk recked no more of men that died than nowadays they would of goats; whereby it very manifestly appeared that that which the natural course of things had not availed, by dint of small and infrequent harms, to teach the wise to endure with patience, the very greatness of their ills had brought even the simple to expect and make no account of. The consecrated ground sufficing not to the burial of the vast multitude of corpses aforesaid, which daily and well nigh hourly came carried in crowds to every church—especially if it were sought to give each his own place, according to ancient usance—there were made throughout the churchyards, after every other part was full, vast trenches, wherein those who came after were laid by the hundred and being heaped up therein by layers, as goods are stored aboard ship, were covered with a little earth, till such time as they reached the top of the trench.

Moreover—not to go longer searching out and recalling every particular of our past miseries, as they befell throughout the city—I say that, whilst so sinister a time prevailed in the latter, on no way therefor was the surrounding country spared, wherein (letting be the castles, which in their littleness were like unto the city) throughout the scattered villages and in the fields, the poor and miserable husbandmen and their families, without succor of physician or aid of servitor, died, not like men, but well nigh like beasts, by the ways or in their tillages or about the houses, indifferently by day and night. By reason whereof, growing lax like the townsfolk in their manners and customs, they recked not of any thing or business of theirs; nay, all, as if they looked for death that very day, studied with all their wit, not to help to maturity the future produce of their cattle and their fields and the fruits of their own past toils, but to consume those which were ready to hand. Thus it came to pass that the oxen, the asses, the sheep, the goats, the swine, the fowls, nay, the very dogs, so faithful to mankind, being driven forth of their own houses, went straying at their pleasure about the fields, where the very grain was abandoned, without being cut, much less gathered in; and many, well nigh like reasonable creatures, after grazing all day, returned at night, glutted, to their houses, without the constraint of any herdsman.

To leave the country and return to the city, what more can be said save that such and so great was the cruelty of heaven (and in part, perhaps, that of men) that, between March and the following July, what with the virulence of that pestiferous sickness and the number of sick ill-tended or forsaken in their need, through the fearfulness of those who were well, it is believed for certain that upward of an hundred thousand human beings perished within the walls of the city of Florence, which, peradventure, before the advent of that death-dealing calamity, had not been believed to hold so many? Alas, how many great palaces, how many goodly houses, how many noble mansions once full of families, of lords and of ladies, abode empty even to the meanest servant! How many memorable families, how many ample heritages, how many famous fortunes were seen to remain without lawful heir! How many valiant men, how many fair ladies, how many sprightly youths, whom, not others only, but Galen, Hippocrates or Aesculapius themselves, would have judged most hale, breakfasted in the morning with their kinsfolk, comrades and friends and that same night supped with their ancestors in the other world!

For the years 1300 to 1351 the chronicle of AGNOLO DI TURA DEL GRASSO ("the Fat") is far more accurate than often is thought to be true of medieval chronicles. The author frequently consulted public records in government archives and offices, and he wrote of the plague of 1348 with the zeal and dedication of one who "buried my five children with my own hands.*

Agnolo di Tura del Grasso

Plague in Siena: An Italian Chronicle

The mortality began in Siena in May [1348]. It was a cruel and horrible thing; and I do not know where to begin to tell of the cruelty and the pitiless ways. It seemed to almost everyone that one became stupified by seeing the pain. And it is impossible for the human tongue to recount the awful thing. Indeed one who did not see such horribleness can be called blessed. And the victims died almost immediately. They would swell beneath their armpits and in their groins, and fall over dead while talking. Father abandoned child, wife husband, one brother another; for this illness seemed to strike through the breath and sight. And so they died. And none could be found to bury the dead for money or friendship. Members of a household brought their dead to a ditch as best they could, without priest, without divine offices. Nor did the death bell sound. And in many places in Siena great pits were dug and piled deep with the multitide of dead. And they died by the hundreds both day and night, and all were thrown in those ditches and covered over with earth. And as soon as those ditches were filled more were dug.

And I, Agnolo di Tura, called the Fat, buried my five children with my own hands. And there were also those who were so sparsely covered with earth that the dogs dragged them forth and devoured many bodies throughout the city.

*From *Cronaca senese attribuita ad Agnolo di Tura del Grasso detta la Cronica Maggiore* in A. Lisini and F. Iacometti (eds.), *Cronache senesi. Rerum Italicarum Scriptores,* n.s. vol. XV, pt. VI (Bologna, 1931–1937), pp. 555, 556, 557, 560. Reprinted by permission of Nicola Zanichelli Editore. Translated by William M. Bowsky.

There was no one who wept for any death, for all awaited death. And so many died that all believed that it was the end of the world. And no medicine or any other defense availed. And the lords[1] selected three citizens who received a thousand gold florins from the commune of Siena that they were to spend on the poor sick and to bury the poor dead. And it was all so horrible that I, the writer, cannot think of it and so will not continue. This situation continued until September, and it would take too long to write of it. And it is found that at this time there died in Siena 36,000 persons twenty years of age or less, and the aged and other people [died], to a total of 52,000 in all in Siena. And in the suburbs of Siena 28,000 persons died; so that in all it is found that in the city and suburbs of Siena 80,000 persons died. Thus at this time Siena and its suburbs had more than 30,000 men, and there remained in Siena [alone] less than 10,000 men.[2] And those that survived were like persons distraught and almost without feeling. And many walls and other things were abandoned, and all the mines of silver and gold and copper that existed in Sienese territory were abandoned as is seen; for in the country-side (contado)[3] many more people died, many lands and villages were abandoned, and no one remained there. I will not write of the cruelty that there was in the countryside, of the wolves and wild beasts that ate the poorly buried corpses, and of other cruelties that would be too painful to those who read of them. . . .

The city of Siena seemed almost uninhabited for almost no one was found in the city. And then, when the pestilence abated, all who survived gave themselves over to pleasures: monks, priests, nuns, and lay men and women all enjoyed themselves, and none worried about spending and gambling. And everyone thought himself rich because he had escaped and regained the world, and no one knew how to allow himself to do nothing. . . .

At this time in Siena the great and noble project of enlarging the cathedral of Siena that had been begun a few years earlier was abandoned. . . .

After the pestilence the Sienese appointed two judges and three non-Sienese notaries whose task it was to handle the wills that had been made at that time. And so they searched them out and found them. . . .

1349.   After the great pestilence of the past year each person lived according to his own caprice, and everyone tended to seek pleasure in eating and drinking, hunting, catching birds, and gaming. And all money had fallen into the hands of *nouveaux riches.*

---

[1] This refers to the lords Nine Governors and Defenders of the Commune and People of Siena, the leading Sienese magistracy from 1287 to 1355.—Ed.

[2] It is not surprising for Agnolo to distinguish between "persons" and "men" (adult males), especially as he relied in large part upon contemporary official documents.—Ed.

[3] The contado of an Italian commune was the portion of the state outside of the city and its boroughs (and in some cases certain adjacent small communities) that was most fully subject to communal jurisdiction.—Ed.

Of peasant stock, JEAN DE VENETTE (d. *ca.* 1368)
became a master of theology at the University of Paris.
He was for several years prior of the Carmelite
monastery in Paris and then head of that order in
France. A good churchman and Frenchman, he was
a careful observer of events that he recorded. The
portion of his chronicle dealing with the Black Death
seems to have been written from memory about a
decade later.*

Jean de Venette

The Chronicle of a French Cleric

1348   In A.D. 1348, the people of France
and of almost the whole world were struck
by a blow other than war. For in addition
to the famine . . . and to the wars . . .
pestilence and its attendant tribulations
appeared again in various parts of the
world. In the month of August, 1348,
after Vespers when the sun was beginning
to set, a big and very bright star appeared
above Paris, toward the west. It did not
seem, as stars usually do, to be very high
above our hemisphere but rather very
near. As the sun set and night came on,
this star did not seem to me or to many
other friars who were watching it to move
from one place. At length, when night
had come, this big star, to the amazement
of all of us who were watching, broke into
many different rays and, as it shed these
rays over Paris toward the east, totally
disappeared and was completely anni-
hilated. Whether it was a comet or not,
whether it was composed of airy exhala-
tions and was finally resolved into vapor,
I leave to the decision of astronomers.
It is, however, possible that it was a pres-
age of the amazing pestilence to come,
which, in fact, followed very shortly in
Paris and throughout France and elsewhere, as I shall tell. All this year and
the next, the mortality of men and wom-
en, of the young even more than of the
old, in Paris and in the kingdom of
France, and also, it is said, in other parts
of the world, was so great that it was almost impossible to bury the dead. People

*From Richard A. Newhall (ed.), *The Chronicle of Jean de Venette,* translated by Jean Birdsall. Records
of Civilization, Sources and Studies, no. 50. Copyright 1953, Columbia University Press, New York. Pp. 48–52.
Footnotes omitted.

lay ill little more than two or three days and died suddenly, as it were in full health. He who was well one day was dead the next and being carried to his grave. Swellings appeared suddenly in the armpit or in the groin—in many cases both—and they were infallible signs of death. This sickness or pestilence was called an epidemic by the doctors. Nothing like the great numbers who died in the years 1348 and 1349 has been heard of or seen or read of in times past. This plague and disease came from *ymaginatione* or association and contagion, for if a well man visited the sick he only rarely evaded the risk of death. Wherefore in many towns timid priests withdrew, leaving the exercise of their ministry to such of the religious as were more daring. In many places not two out of twenty remained alive. So high was the mortality at the Hôtel-Dieu[1] in Paris that for a long time, more than five hundred dead were carried daily with great devotion in carts to the cemetery of the Holy Innocents in Paris for burial. A very great number of the saintly sisters of the Hôtel-Dieu who, not fearing to die, nursed the sick in all sweetness and humility, with no thought of honor, a number too often renewed by death, rest in peace with Christ, as we may piously believe.

This plague, it is said, began among the unbelievers, came to Italy, and then crossing the Alps reached Avignon, where it attacked several cardinals and took from them their whole household. Then it spread, unforeseen, to France, through Gascony and Spain, little by little, from town to town, from village to village, from house to house, and finally from person to person. It even crossed over to Germany, though it was not so bad there as with us. During the epidemic, God of His accustomed goodness deigned to grant this grace, that however suddenly men died, almost all awaited death joyfully. Nor was there anyone who died without confessing his sins and receiving the holy viaticum.[2] To the even greater benefit of the dying, Pope Clement VI through their confessors mercifully gave and granted absolution from penalty to the dying in many cities and fortified towns. Men died the more willingly for this and left many inheritances and temporal goods to churches and monastic orders, for in many cases they had seen their close heirs and children die before them.

Some said that this pestilence was caused by infection of the air and waters, since there was at this time no famine nor lack of food supplies, but on the contrary great abundance. As a result of this theory of infected water and air as the source of the plague the Jews were suddenly and violently charged with infecting wells and water and corrupting the air. The whole world rose up against them cruelly on this account. In Germany and other parts of the world where Jews lived, they were massacred and slaughtered by Christians, and many thousands were burned everywhere, indiscriminately. The unshaken, if fatuous, constancy of the men and their wives was remarkable. For mothers hurled their children first into the fire that they might not be baptized and then leaped in after them to burn with their husbands and children. It is said that many bad Christians were found who in a like manner put poison into wells. But in truth, such poisonings, granted that they actually were perpetrated, could not have caused so great a plague nor have infected so many people. There were other causes; for example, the will of God

---

[1] The principal hospital.—Ed.

[2] The viaticum is the Eucharist, or Communion, given to the dying.—Ed.

and the corrupt humors and evil inherent in air and earth. Perhaps the poisonings, if they actually took place in some localities, reenforced these causes. The plague lasted in France for the greater part of the years 1348 and 1349 and then ceased. Many country villages and many houses in good towns remained empty and deserted. Many houses, including some splendid dwellings, very soon fell into ruins. Even in Paris several houses were thus ruined, though fewer here than elsewhere.

After the cessation of the epidemic, pestilence, or plague, the men and women who survived married each other. There was no sterility among the women, but on the contrary fertility beyond the ordinary. Pregnant women were seen on every side. Many twins were born and even three children at once. But the most surprising fact is that children born after the plague, when they became of an age for teeth, had only twenty or twenty-two teeth, though before that time men commonly had thirty-two in their upper and lower jaws together. What this diminution in the number of teeth signified I wonder greatly, unless it be a new era resulting from the destruction of one human generation by the plague and its replacement by another. But woe is me! the world was not changed for the better but for the worse by this renewal of population. For men were more avaricious and grasping than before, even though they had far greater possessions. They were more covetous and disturbed each other more frequently with suits, brawls, disputes, and pleas. Nor by the mortality resulting from this terrible plague inflicted by God was peace between kings and lords established. On the contrary, the enemies of the king of France and of the Church were stronger and wickeder than before and stirred up wars on sea and on land. Great-

er evils than before pullulated everywhere in the world. And this fact was very remarkable. Although there was an abundance of all goods, yet everything was twice as dear, whether it were utensils, victuals, or merchandise, hired helpers or peasants and serfs, except for some hereditary domains which remained abundantly stocked with everything. Charity began to cool, and iniquity with ignorance and sin to abound, for few could be found in the good towns and castles who knew how or were willing to instruct children in the rudiments of grammar. . . .

1349 In the year 1349, while the plague was still active and spreading from town to town, men in Germany, Flanders, Hainaut, and Lorraine uprose and began a new sect on their own authority. Stripped to the waist, they gathered in large groups and bands and marched in procession through the crossroads and squares of cities and good towns. There they formed circles and beat upon their backs with weighted scourges, rejoicing as they did so in loud voices and singing hymns suitable to their rite and newly composed for it. Thus for thirty-three days they marched through many towns doing their penance and affording a great spectacle to the wondering people. They flogged their shoulders and arms with scourges tipped with iron points so zealously as to draw blood. But they did not come to Paris nor to any part of France, for they were forbidden to do so by the king of France, who did not want them. He acted on the advice of the masters of theology of the University of Paris, who said that this new sect had been formed contrary to the will of God, to the rites of Holy Mother Church, and to the salvation of all their souls. That indeed this was and is true appeared shortly. For Pope

Clement VI was fully informed concerning this fatuous new rite by the masters of Paris through emissaries reverently sent to him and, on the grounds that it had been damnably formed, contrary to law, he forbade the Flagellants under threat of anathema to practise in the future the public penance which they had so presumptuously undertaken. His prohibition was just, for the Flagellants, supported by certain fatuous priests and monks, were enunciating doctrines and opinions which were beyond measure evil, erroneous, and fallacious. For example, they said that their blood thus drawn by the scourge and poured out was mingled with the blood of Christ. Their many errors showed how little they knew of the Catholic faith. Wherefore, as they had begun fatuously of themselves and not of God, so in a short time they were reduced to nothing. On being warned, they desisted and humbly received absolution and penance at the hands of their prelates as the pope's representatives. Many honorable women and devout matrons, it must be added, had done this penance with scourges, marching and singing through towns and churches like the men, but after a little like the others they desisted.

JAMES WESTFALL THOMPSON (1869–1941) was long
a professor of history at the University of Chicago.
His numerous published works include *Economic and
Social History of the Middle Ages* and *Feudal
Germany,* both published in 1928, and *A History of
Historical Writing,* which appeared posthumously.
The change in his interests from largely political to
social, economic, and cultural history was presaged
in his provocative article on the Black Death.*

James Westfall Thompson

The Plague and World War:
Parallels and Comparisons

Ever since the Great War terminated
and the world lapsed into the condition —
physical, moral, economic, social — in
which it now finds itself, historians and
students of social pathology have been
searching if possibly they might discover
a precedent in the past for the present
order (or rather disorder) of things. The
years immediately following the close
of the Napoleonic Wars have been the
favorite epoch for examination. But the
conditions of the period after Waterloo
have been found to bear little resemblance
to conditions today. The differences in
degree between things as they were then
and things as they now are is so great
that analogies fail. The old maxims, "We
understand the present by the past," and
"History is philosophy teaching by
example," are broken shibboleths. There
seems to have been nothing in the past
comparable or applicable to the present.

And yet, though it is true that history
never repeats itself, there is one epoch
of the past the study of which casts remarkable light upon things as they are
today; whose conditions afford phenom-
enal parallels in many particulars to
present conditions; which furnishes not
merely analogies but real identities with
existing economic, social, and moral
circumstances. That period is the years
immediately succeeding the Great Plague
or the Black Death of 1348–49 in Europe.

---

*From James Westfall Thompson, "The Aftermath of the Black Death and the Aftermath of the Great
War," *The American Journal of Sociology,* XXVI (1921), 565–572, published by The University of Chicago
Press.

The turmoil of the world today serves to visualize for us what the state of Europe was in the middle of the fourteenth century far more distinctly than ever was perceived before. It is surprising to see how similar are the complaints then and now: economic chaos, social unrest, high prices, profiteering, depravation of morals, lack of production, industrial indolence, frenetic gaiety, wild expenditure, luxury, debauchery, social and religious hysteria, greed, avarice, maladministration, decay of manners.

Let us consider the first and most immediate effect—the loss of man-power owing to the great mortality. While it is true that the population of Europe is much greater now than in the fourteenth century, and the mortality far higher then than in the past five years, nevertheless, as everyone knows, the working efficiency of Europe has been seriously reduced owing to the death of large numbers of men in battle or of disease, to which must be added some millions of the civilian population from starvation, privation, and disease. And many of those who survive are shaken in body or in mind. The nerves of these people are so shattered that it will be a long time before they can go back to work; many of them never will. The same was true of the people of Europe in 1349, when the Black Death had passed. The psycho-physical shock to them had been so great that restoration of their former vitality and initiative was impossible, or very slow.

The economic effect of the Black Death also was not unsimilar to the effect of the Great War, though the immediate results of the plague were very different. The moment the war began prices soared. This was not so in 1349. The immediate effect of the Black Death was to lower prices and to glut the market with commodities. The reason is not far to seek.

Every civilized society possesses a certain accumulated surplus of goods or produce, enough to last it for some months at least, even if production cease. Now the mortality due to the Black Death was very high, at least 35 per cent of the population. The consequence was that when the plague had spent its force the surviving population found itself in possession of these accumulated stores, produce, goods, in addition to movable and real property which had once belonged to those now dead.

Men woke up to find themselves rich who had formerly been poor, inasmuch as they were the only surviving heirs. Land, houses, furniture, goods, farm products, cattle, horses, sheep, were without owners, and most of it was immediately appropriated by the survivors. Everything movable or which could be driven away on four feet was seized; even landed property was occupied since there was no one to protest and the very courts of law were stopped. "There were small prices for everything," records Henry Knighton, the medieval chronicler. "A man could have a horse, which before was worth 40s. for 6s. 8d.; a fat ox for 4s.; a cow for 12d.; a heifer for 2d.; a big pig for 5d.; a fat wether for 4d.; a sheep for 3d.; a lamb for 2d.; a stone of wool for 9d. Sheep and cattle went wandering over fields and through crops, and there was no one to go and drive or gather them."

The direct result of all this suddenly acquired wealth was a wild orgy of expenditure and debauchery on the part of many. Furs, silks, tapestries, rich furniture, expensive food, jewels, plate, fell within the purchasing power of the poor. Men spent lavishly, luxuriously, insanely. Poor workmen and poorer cotters, living in wretched hovels, who formerly, like Margery Daw, had slept on straw, now lolled on beds of down and ate from plate that once had decorated the sideboards of nobles. Often, too, they removed from their ancient quarters into the vacant houses. The landlord class was hit hard by the plague. "Magnates and lesser lords of the realm who had tenants made abatements of rent in order to keep their tenantry; some half the rent, some more, some less, some for two years, some for three, some for one year, according as they could agree with them."

But this condition of luxury soon passed. Those who survived found themselves personally richer than before; but Europe was immeasurably poorer, for production absolutely ceased for months, even a whole year, and when it was renewed the productive capacity of Europe was found to be much impaired, while the waste had been terrific. When all the accumulated surplus had been consumed or wasted, prices soared and the cost of living, both of commodities and of service, rose enormously. Farm laborers, guild workmen, domestic servants, clerks, even priests, struck for higher wages. "In the following autumn no one could get a reaper for less than 8*d*. with his food; a mower for less than 12*d*. with his food. Wherefore many crops perished in the fields for want of some one to garner them. But in the pestilence year there was such abundance of all kinds of corn that no one troubled about it. . . . A man could scarcely get a chaplain under ten pounds or ten marks to minister to a church. There was scarcely any one now who was willing to accept a vicarage for twenty pounds." Even rents soon went up. Abandoned buildings lapsed into ruin, occupied buildings naturally deteriorated under wear and tear, and the wages of carpenters and other artisans were often so high as to prohibit repairs.

The high prices of staple commodities and the exorbitant demands of the wage-earning class soon reached a pinnacle under the stimulus of profiteering. Accordingly the governments had resort to maximum laws both for commodities and wages. France passed a Statute of Laborers in 1350, England a similar law in 1351.

The social effects of the Black Death were manifold. In the first place, then as now, there was enormous displacement of population. The plague had the effect of an invasion; it either killed or drove out the population. Thousands fled to other places. Infected districts were left deserted. In after-years one finds evidence of this in interesting ways. New place-names, new faces, even unfamiliar speech in various regions, attest it. One finds evidence of Italian colonies in south German and south French cities; French and Germans in north Italy; Flemings in Normandy; Normans in Picardy, etc. Under the stress of fear men were mad to get out of an infected region, and fled, often into another quite as dangerous. We find other evidence of this movement of population in the outcropping of technical industries and crafts, once peculiar to a certain country, in quite another place owing to the flight of workmen from the former to the latter locality.

The texture of society, too, was profoundly modified by the Black Death. In addition to a large class of *nouveaux riches,* the plague opened the door of opportunity to many to get into new lines of employment, or to establish themselves in new kinds of business. Clerks became merchants, former workmen became employers and contractors, farm laborers became gentlemen farmers. The old nobility of Europe, which derived its lineage from the Norman Conquest and the Crusades, largely passed away, leaving their titles and their lands to the kings who gave them out to new favorites, so that a new *noblesse* arose in Europe, a parvenu nobility without the accomplishment, the pride, or the manners of the old *noblesse*. The titles survived, but the blood of the peerage was new, not old; parvenu, not aristocratic. With the passing of the aristocracy passed also the chivalry and courtesy that had distinguished it. The decay of manners in the last half of the fourteenth century is an astonishing fact. The old-fashioned gentility was gone; manners were uncouth, rough, brutal. Familiar speech became rude, lewd, even obscene. Every student of the literature of the fourteenth and fifteenth centuries has observed this. This explains the paradox that books on courtesy were so much in demand in these centuries. The new high society was ignorant of good manners and needed to know. Even fashions reflected the decadent conditions of the age. Refinement and decorum in dress, which marked the distinguished lady and gentleman in the thirteenth century, disappeared. The *nouveaux riches* had a passion for display, for garish colors, for excessive dress, for the wearing of many jewels. Dressmakers and milliners reaped a harvest from this class. The costumes were fabrications to wonder at, but not to admire.

Another characteristic of the late fourteenth century which strikes a familiar note is the protest against political corruption and administrative inefficiency. The cry for reform was widespread and not to be wondered at. The Black Death hit the governments of Europe hard. For two hundred years these governments had been slowly and painfully developing their administrative machinery and training up a skilled class of officials in their employ. Now of a sudden thousands of this technically trained class were cut down, so much so that the governments were crippled beyond what we may imagine; police protection, courts, law-making, the hundred and one everyday activities of an ordered society were arrested. The machinery of the governments nearly stopped. In this emergency two things happened: the offices had to be filled, the government kept running at all cost, so that thousands of ignorant, incompetent, dishonest men were hastily thrust into public offices; moreover, the thousands of vacant offices tempted the jobhunter, the placemen, the professional office-seeker, and this class swarmed into the vacancies with the selfish motive of feathering their own nests and plundering the public. The result was appalling waste, great maladministration, peculation, etc., with the natural protest of society against these abuses.

The church was no better off than the state in this particular. Every student of medieval history knows the outcry that arose in Europe in the last half of the fourteenth century against the abuses and corruption in the church. But the church is not to be blamed too severely for this condition. It, too, had to keep functioning, and to do so impressed into service all sorts and conditions of men; in the universal terror it could not be over-careful in those whom it selected. And again, church offices were lucrative and influential appointments, and many intruded themselves into church livings for the sake of the material nature of the preferment.

Complaints against political and administrative corruption, the prevalence and increase of crime, lightness of mind, and looseness of morals, high prices, profiteering, industrial and farm strikes, extravagance, indolence, or refusal to go to work are common and widespread today. So they were in the fourteenth century. The Black Death wrought a universal upheaval and transformation of society to which nothing else in history is comparable except the influence of the Great War.

Even in the field of psychology this analogy holds true. Not only those who actually fought in the late war, but the whole population is suffering from "shell shock," from frayed nerves. It is this condition which explains the semi-hysterical state of mind of millions in Europe, which accounts for their fevered or morbid emotionalism. The old barriers are down, the old inhibitions removed. The superficial yet fevered gaiety, the proneness to debauchery, the wild wave of extravagance, the flamboyant luxury, the gluttony in restaurant and café—all these phenomena are readily explicable by the student used to making psycho-social analyses. And as always at such seasons, the phenomena of the Freudian complex are vividly presented. A book could be written solely upon the strange, intense, morbid sex manifestations abroad in the world at present.

It was so after the Black Death. The so-called Flagellant movement was a mixture of religious morbidity and sex stimuli, so widespread in its influence that it reduced thousands to a state of frenzy. Not since the Crusades had Europe witnessed so tremendous a manifestation of mob psychology. In the lapse of all the accustomed inhibitions of church, of state, of society, the thought and conduct of men went off on eccentric tangents. The failure of old authorities gave room for new and self-constituted authorities to establish themselves. Charlatans, mind-readers, sorcerers, witch-doctors, drug-vendors, sprang up like mushrooms, along with perfervid crossroads preachers and soap-box orators

denouncing society and the wrongs around them, and offering each his panacea or remedy. A golden opportunity was afforded to the amateur preacher, the amateur reformer, the pseudo-scientist, the grafter.

The literature of the late Middle Ages is rich in the possession of this kind of psycho-social phenomena, which has not yet been studied. Few even know of it. It may surprise the reader to learn that probably the well-known legend about the Pied Piper of Hamelin is attached to the time of the Black Death. Grotesque and amusing as Browning's famous ballad is, there is yet a tragic pathos underneath the tale, which he failed to divine. Browning, as all his readers, regarded the story as a mere legend. But undeniably there is a basis of real history below the surface.

In the first place it is a well-known historical fact that the Black Death was accompanied by a great plague of rats in Europe. Now the rat has been a symbol of pestilence since remote antiquity. One need go no farther than the Old Testament for evidence of this, and the symbolism is attested by ancient art. What probably happened at Hamelin was this: the town was infested by rats; the Pied Piper made his appearance (whether a charlatan or a lunatic cannot be said) and offered to charm the rats away. The rats probably stayed, but the Piper's strange costume and stranger power which he declared that he possessed, united with the intense, even hysterical emotionalism of the people, working upon the natural curiosity of children at sight of such a wondrous spectacle as the Piper in their streets, lured the children after him and they were scattered, never to return. The poor children were swept away on a wave of crowd psychology, of emotional excitement, to the point of hysteria. They suffered the fate of those who went on the Children's Crusade, many of whom we know fell into the hands of professional kidnappers and slavers.

A book might be written upon these peculiar and eccentric effects of the Black Death, as many will write books in the near future upon the social psychology of Europe since the war. The parallel which I have made is not a perfect one, of course, but there is sufficient analogy between the aftermath of the Black Death and the aftermath of the Great War to enlist the serious consideration of the student of history.

YVES RENOUARD (1908–1965), professor at the University of Bordeaux and later at the Sorbonne, was a specialist in the economic and social history of the later Middle Ages. He worked for many years in Rome and Florence, and his best-known study is a scholarly volume on the relations of the Avignon popes with banking and commercial companies from 1316 to 1378. That he also could write for educated nonspecialists is amply demonstrated by his short books on the Avignon papacy (1954), the history of Florence (1964), and Italian businessmen (1949). The same skill is evident in his lucid and wide-ranging article on the impact of the Black Death.*

Yves Renouard

The Black Death as a Major Event in World History

The Black Death of 1348, because of its universal nature, the demographic collapse it caused throughout the Western and Mediterranean world, and its profound effect on all facets of life, was probably the most important event of fourteenth-century history. . . .

Epidemics were frequent in the Middle Ages. Efforts to combat them effectively were hindered by lack of hygiene and the inadequacies of medical science. On the average one could expect a serious or even disastrous epidemic every quarter-century.

Many epidemics first appeared in the great urban centers of the Near and Middle East, where a number of diseases are still endemic. Caravans and ships then spread them abroad. We do not know exactly where or how, in 1347, the Black Death began. The first manifestation of the plague appeared in the great Genoese colony of Kaffa in the Crimea, on the shores of the Black Sea. Janibeg, the Mongol khan of the Kipchaks besieged this port, which was easily supplied by sea. When an epidemic of the plague broke out in his army, he used catapults to hurl the dead into the town. He did this not only to rid himself of the bodies, but also in the hope that the plague would spread among the besieged, weakening their resistance. Here, with this simple operation, we already have chemical warfare.

Actually, Janibeg's scheme failed; he

*From Yves Renouard, "La Peste Noire de 1348–50," *La Revue de Paris*, LVII (March, 1950), 107–119. Translated by William M. Bowsky. Footnotes omitted.

was unable to take Kaffa. The defenders greatly limited the spread of the contagion by immediately throwing into the sea the corpses with which they were bombarded, and they were able to resist. But it was enough that some fell ill and that after the siege certain of these returned to the west for the "Black Death" to spread rapidly.

The disease only later received the name Black Death from the dark-colored blemishes that developed on the limbs of the sick. Without doubt it was the bubonic plague, characterized by the swelling of tumors, or buboes, on the arms and groin, a gangrenous inflammation of the throat and lungs, violent chest pains, vomiting and spitting blood, and the stench of the victim's body.

It was spread by objects touched by the sick as well as by direct contact. The suddenness and rapidity of the disease were such that a subject could pass from perfect health to death in one day. Generally the illness lasted only from three to five days, during the course of which the patient was overcome by fever and tortured by an intense thirst. . . .

In the space of two and a half years the Black Death traversed the whole of Europe. It was not that men failed to try to halt its advance or at least protect themselves from it. All the physicians of the time were concerned with the plague. A highly esteemed Italian doctor, Gentile da Foligno, renowned for his teaching at Padua, wrote *Consilia contra pestilentiam* [Treatises against the pestilence]; but he died in June 1348, a victim of his devotion to the sick, who had pressed around him. At Montpellier, where the university was famous for the skill of its medical faculty, all the doctors died of the plague. When the plague neared Paris, King Philip VI sought advice from the Paris Faculty of Medicine. It produced a *Com-*

pendium de epidemia per collegium Facultatis medicorum Parisius ordinatum [Compendium concerning the epidemic composed by the College of the Paris Faculty of Medicine] which remains outstanding. But it was a descriptive rather than a therapeutic work.

Nevertheless, the plague continued its inexorable progress toward the north. Before it reached the gates of Reims, Pierre de Damouzy, a doctor from Champagne, composed an interesting treatise on its prevention. He began by explaining that the fact that the plague struck some and spared others was due to the influence of the stars. But he went on to give some practical advice on how to avoid infection. He repeated Rhazes'[1] old prescription: to protect himself from the plague a person should stay at home with doors and windows shut; if he absolutely has to go out, he should carry camphor, amber, or some other disinfectant. Further, Damouzy recommended bleeding, purging, and a lightened diet; he absolutely forbade bathing and lovemaking. Although many of his prescriptions seemed sensible and judicious, the plague continued to spread.

The spread of the Black Death marked the complete failure of contemporary medicine. It also showed the futility of conceiving of charity and religion as a prophylaxis. Some religious orders were tirelessly devoted to the care of plague victims, but they saved only a very small number of the sick, and many religious brotherhoods lost their entire memberships. Ecclesiastical authorities instituted suitable prayers; Pope Clement VI established a special office to win God's mercy.

---

[1] Rhazes or al Rāzī (*ca.* 865–924) was a great Persian Muslim physician who wrote numerous valuable treatises on a variety of subjects. His major medical work, "Comprehensive Book," was translated into Latin in the thirteenth century.—Ed.

This was largely in vain, just as it was in vain for popular piety to turn to Saint Sebastian, Saint Anthony, and Saint Adrian, holy protectors who were reputed to fight epidemics.

The blind barbarity that turned the wrath of the credulous masses against the Jews had no more success. The Jews were accused of spreading the epidemic by poisoning wells. They were persecuted everywhere, but it was particularly in Spain that terror of the plague stirred up the flames of anti-Semitism. At Avignon, the Pope protected the Jews from all violence.

The only preventive measure that had any efficacy was, by definition, the tactic of cowards. Those who were able to flee to a healthy part of the countryside, far from population centers, before they were infected succeeded in escaping the plague. But this was a rich man's defense, available especially to kings, princes, and lords. After having shown a great deal of courage Pope Clement VI finally withdrew to Villeneuve-les-Avignon. Many rich bourgeois also had recourse to this defense, witness the eight young women and two young men of the *Decameron,* who sought amusement and health in a villa in the Tuscan hills.

Thus, despite practical and scholarly cures, despite prayer and popular wrath, men all over Europe continued to die. The number of dead was such that contemporaries viewed the epidemic as an unprecedented disaster.

Boccaccio estimates that more than a hundred thousand died in Florence; a chronicler of Rouen gives the same number for that city, and Gilles li Muisit notes twenty-five thousand for Tournai. Froissart devoted only one sentence of his long work to the plague, but it has become famous: "In this time a disease which is called an epidemic raged generally throughout the world, and a good third of the world died of it." Simon de Couvin of Montpellier estimates that the plague carried off half the population.

These figures are clearly exaggerated; those given for towns even exceed the total number of their inhabitants. Moreover, if a third or half of the total population had perished, Europe would have become a kind of wasteland. But events after 1350 testify that a dense population still existed.

The plague did not strike all regions, all human groupings, and all social categories with the same intensity. As was to be expected, population centers were particularly hard hit. The towns, where hygiene was deplorable, suffered much more than the countryside. And in the towns social groups that lived crowded together, such as members of the working class and friars of the mendicant orders, suffered most.

Surviving archival documents give us an accurate idea of the size of the mortality in certain instances. Study of the accounts of the Apostolic Chamber reveals that 94 persons probably died of the *infirmitias* [plague] at the pontifical court of Avignon in 1348–1349. Since the court had a total of 450 members, this represents nearly a fourth.

The parish register kept by the pastor of the village of Givry, near Chalon-sur-Saône in Burgundy, has been preserved for the period of the epidemic. In the preceding decade an average of 30 persons died annually in this prosperous village of 1200 to 1500 inhabitants; but from August 5 to November 19, 1348, 615 persons died, almost half the population. The calculations for the English clergy made by Gasquet[2] suggest that

[2] The Benedictine Cardinal, Francis Aidan Gasquet, whose *The Great Pestilence* was published in 1893. — Ed.

between 1348 and 1350 nearly half were lost to the plague. Doren[3] estimates that in Italy from 40 to 60 percent of the urban population perished, but that the losses were much less in the countryside. Certain evidence seems to confirm this urban hecatomb: For example, the commune of Siena had undertaken the construction of an immense and splendid cathedral, of which the old cathedral would have constituted only a transept, but the plague interrupted the work. The depopulation and ruin of the town made it useless and impossible to resume construction. On the immense esplanade that surrounds the cathedral of Siena, the black and white columns of this projected edifice still reach heavenward in unhappy, mournful appeal.

But the worst losses known are those suffered by the monasteries of the mendicant orders. The Dominican monasteries of Tuscany and Languedoc[4] did not always have as many as a hundred friars each; those such as Santa Maria Novella at Florence which had more than 150 were quite rare. When the plague struck, 78 friars died in Florence, 49 in Siena, 57 in Pisa, and 39 in Lucca. There remained only 7 out of 140 at Montpellier and 7 of 160 at Maguelonne. In the monasteries of the Cordeliers, at Marseille and Carcassonne, all the friars died. Thus the proportion of plague deaths in relation to the total population seems to have oscillated from a half to an eighth according to the region.

These innumerable victims were not all persons without significance. Some had made names for themselves in certain human endeavor. Strangers to each other, differing in age, they were bound together by a common date of death. There were kings and princes among them. The son of the Byzantine emperor, Andronicus Comnenus, died in three days at Constantinople; Leonora of Portugal (Queen of Aragon), Princess Maria of Aragon (daughter of King Peter IV's first marriage), the Count and Countess of Ribagorce, and King Alfonso XI of Castile also were taken by the plague. Edward III's daughter Joan of England, who was the fiancée of Peter the Cruel, son and successor of Alfonso XI, died in Bordeaux in August 1348, on the way to her future kingdom. Some celebrated prelates and theologians also perished. Among them were two successive archbishops of Canterbury; the second, Thomas Bradwardine, was one of the most learned masters of the University of Oxford. Also in this category were the Augustinian monk Simone Fidati da Cascia, renowned for his *De gestis Domini Salvatoris,* the first life of Christ written since the Gospels, and Cardinal Giovanni Colonna, Petrarch's[5] friend and protector, who died at Avignon on July 3, 1348. Three months earlier, in the first days of April, Petrarch's inspiration, Laura de Noves, was carried off by the plague. Petrarch, then absent at Parma, learned simultaneously of the deaths of the two persons he cherished most. In the famous verse in which he mourns them, he associates the memory of the mistress of his heart with that of his patron:

Broken is the tall column and green laurel which shaded my weary thought.

Among artists, the two Sienese painters Ambrogio and Pietro Lorenzetti, who had decorated the principal buildings of Siena with their frescoes, the Florentine painter

---

[3] Alfred J. Doren, a German economic historian who specialized in Italian economic history.—Ed.
[4] Southern France—Ed.

[5] Francesco Petrarca (1304–74), an early Italian humanist.—Ed.

Bernardo Daddi, one of Giotto's best pupils, and the sculptor Andrea Pisano succumbed in 1348. Among businessmen, Giovanni Villani, associated first with the Florentine Peruzzi company, later with the Buonaccorsi, in his exactness and objectivity the greatest chronicler of the fourteenth century, died in 1348, leaving his pen to his brother Matteo. Sir John Pulteney, a member of the Company of Drapers of London, four times mayor, and the greatest banker in the city, was carried off some months later. Among soldiers who died was Sir John Montgomery, the first English captain of recently conquered Calais. And the testaments to many common people mournfully recall their collective deaths.

No weddings took place during the pestilence, but once it seemed over there were unusually many. The parish register of Givry mentions no weddings in 1348, but 86 in 1349, of which 42 took place between January 14 and February 24. And this was among a population reduced to a few hundred inhabitants. Evidently, surviving widowers, whatever their age, remarried with a young man's haste. Guillaume de Nangis's continuator notes this in his chronicle: "At the end of this epidemic, pestilence, and mortality, men and women married each other." It was necessary to restore the hearths in villages where perhaps only one still remained. But however fecund these new unions were, only in time could they remedy the severe demographic setback that the plague had caused throughout the world. For at least a generation Europe was again in that state of underpopulation from which it had wrested itself since the twelfth century.

This swift and unequal demographic collapse following immediately upon the psychological and mental shock caused by the epidemic (during which each person felt himself menaced and lived through frightful hours) had the greatest consequence in all areas.

Frightened by the approach of the plague, which they saw as God's instrument of vengeance for the punishment of their sins, certain men sought to appease divine wrath by penances as exceptional as the plague itself. Thus a preventive movement of mortification and mysticism began in Germany. Men and women assembled and left their homes in bands of several hundred under the leadership of one or more chiefs, whom they called masters in imitation of the mendicant orders. In each locality that they traversed they stopped and publicly whipped themselves with cruel violence while singing laments:

Let us strike our "flesh" [carrion] sharply while remembering the Lord's great passion and his piteous death.

In imitating Christ's passion, these Flagellants sought to obtain God's pardon through the intercession of the Virgin. This mixture of mortification and piety, which well expressed the collective panic of the population, disquieted the authorities. But the mental contagion spread almost as quickly as the contagion it wished to destroy. Before the movement finally ended, the Flagellants had spread to Bohemia and Hungary in the east and to Picardie and Champagne in the west.

The collective mental shock, which reached its high point with the Flagellants, did not spare many of their contemporaries. Fear of the plague and the spectacle of disease and corpses aroused in most persons ideas of penitence and the constant thought of death. The passion of Christ, which the Flagellants wanted to suffer in their own bodies, became a theme of habitual meditation. It is reproduced in scenes that decorate religious edifices and private oratories. Also, the cult of the Five Wounds of Christ became prevalent. The frescoes of the Camposanto of Pisa show how strongly the epidemic turned men's imaginations to the mystery of death. . . . Macabre themes multiplied in the figurative arts.

Only heroes and heroines of romances such as Fiammetta, Pampinea, and their friends[6] had the will and the ability to forget so many scenes of horror while residing in the beautiful gardens to which they had fled, amid dancing, feasting, siestas, and stories that aroused laughter and exalted the joy of living. Some contemporaries reacted against the destroying menace, by which they felt immeasurably burdened, by giving themselves over to sensual pleasures, free of care and with feverish violence. They abandoned themselves to debauchery, gluttonously satisfying all their appetites. During the same period that the mystical crisis we mentioned occurred, a wave of immorality shook the entire West. "After the great pestilence of the past year, each person lived according to his own caprice . . . ," notes the Sienese Agnolo di Tura.

In the countryside as in the towns, the plague carried off proportionally more peasants and workers than lords and bourgeois. Suddenly the supply of labor had dwindled.

On certain English manors all the tenants died. At the beginning of the epidemic, this rural mortality caused the halt of all work in the countryside. In certain areas, such as northern Italy, by the testimony of John of Parma, the harvest of 1348 remained in the fields. The relative abundance of products in relation to the suddenly decimated popula-tion and people's concern simply with living, no longer worrying about gain or the future, caused an initial price drop. But things changed quickly. The peak of the plague passed, and survivors abandoned poor or badly situated land in order to settle on the best land, to which lords attracted them by giving them the concessions they craved: enfranchisment if they were serfs, better conditions of tenure and high wages (wages at least 50 to 100 percent higher than before the plague).

The agrarian structure of the West was considerably disrupted. The system of the seigneurial reserve, which was already declining, disappeared completely in many regions. This was because the peasants tended to cultivate only their own tenures, whose produce they kept for themselves. The lords, both lay and ecclesiastical, suffered an unbelievable diminution in revenue from ground rents. Rents dropped by half, sometimes by three-quarters, because of the immense amount of land that was abandoned and because conditions had become very favorable for tenants on the lands that remained in cultivation. Offerings to churches decreased in the same proportion. The old class of landed proprietors, the nobility and the clergy, had its principal source of power severely shaken; castles, churches, rural monasteries, and even hospitals fell into ruin.

The scarcity of agrarian products and of fish caused their prices to soar; this had grave consequences for the urban population.

In the towns the heavy mortality led to a scarcity of artisanal and industrial labor even greater than the shortage of labor in the countryside. It also caused severe disorganization of local and long-distance commerce, since not only was the local clientele reduced, but nearly all foreign

---

[6] These are the storytellers in Boccaccio's *Decameron.* — Ed.

markets were affected as well. The workers, less numerous and no longer able to subsist because of the rise in food prices, demanded wage increases. The richest artisans profited from the situation by attracting all available laborers into their shops or under their control, thus ruining their competitors. Lesser officials made the same demands as the workers, for the same reasons. In 1349 the trumpeters of the commune of Florence explained to the authorities that they were no longer able to live on their wages. That same year the wax-warmers of the pontifical chancery and other employees of the palace service "no longer wished to work if their salary was not increased."

The scarcity of labor permitted survivors to obtain wage increases that were proportionally perhaps a bit greater than the increases in food prices. Thus the miserable level of their lives was slightly improved. The increase in urban wages varied from 50 to 150 percent, according to the town and the trade.

The ordinances enacted by the authorities in 1351 (especially by the kings of France and England) to hinder workers from quitting their employers and demanding wages higher than those of 1347 remained inoperative. The enactment of such ordinances was demanded primarily by landed proprietors and frightened consumers. Despite the adoption of regulations, those badly adapted to the new circumstances were crushed by the inexorable play of fundamental economic laws.

The crisis caused by the Black Death entailed a definite rise in the price of manufactured goods and the stagnation of commerce. The stagnation of commerce was caused by the sudden loss of some of its clientele. The English merchant companies, which leased their right to export wool from the king, were ruined

in a few months. The king, who wished to use these companies also for borrowing money, was forced to revise his entire economic policy and to receive foreign merchants favorably.

The states of Europe suffered the consequences of these economic disturbances. The numerical decline in population and the ruin of taxpayers caused a drop in revenue which left the principal political nations of the West powerless for a time, just at the moment when their fiscal development allowed them to conceive of great enterprises.

The king of France, the king of England, the pope, and the Italian republics had to renounce temporarily their extensive political and military activities. The plague had made the raising of armies difficult, not only by terrifying the population from which the soldiers must come, but also by causing a decline in the revenue needed to pay them. After the initial success of the Dauphin Humbert's crusade, a truce was concluded between Christians and Saracens in 1348. It was broken only eleven years later after Peter I of Lusignan gained the throne of Cyprus. The threat of war between the two coalitions formed by Venice and Genoa in 1345 did not materialize until 1351, when hostilities began. Finally, after the [French] defeat at Crécy and the loss of Calais the Franco-English conflict was abated by a truce signed in 1347, which was renewed till 1355. Even the civil war in Flanders, caused by the fall of Artevelde in 1346, stopped when the plague entered that country.

Political circumstances do not perhaps alone explain the general abatement of conflicts.

The reduction in revenues which struck the princes caused them to dispute more harshly the revenues they shared. For several decades the English king had been enduring, with difficulty, the intensification of the papal hold on the English clergy. It was significant that after the outbreaks of the plague in 1351 and 1353, Edward III enacted the celebrated statutes against papal conferment of English ecclesiastical benefices and against abuses of the pontifical fisc. The impoverished English clergy was no longer able to pay taxes to both the king and the pope.

In the countryside, a great many ruined nobles took up brigandage, even before the great mercenary companies were formed in France.

The social consequences of the plague were particularly significant in the towns, where men lived more closely together than in the countryside and dealt more constantly with one another. By causing a large number of the bourgeois to perish, the plague allowed the survivors to gain possession of the property of the dead. The Black Death thus created enormous fortunes. The workers and artisans, however, who escaped death inherited only the worn-out clothing of their deceased relatives. While the plague made the rich richer, it left the poor as before; the total wretchedness of the poor continued while the affluence of the rich reached unprecedented levels of opulence. In the urban microcosm the contrast between wealth and poverty became greater than ever before. Patrician ostentation and sumptuousness burst forth even in Florence, where business men were experiencing terrible financial troubles, which since 1342 had caused the successive collapse of all the greatest commercial companies. A great many citizens, after having seen their whole family die, bequeathed all their property to charitable institutions. Thus, the Company of San Michele, to which all the great merchants contributed, increased its patrimony by 350,000

florins. It should have distributed this money to the poor, but taking into consideration that the plague had killed a great many of these, it decided to use part of this sum to construct a tabernacle to shelter the miraculous Madonna, the company's emblem. Andrea Orcagna was charged with constructing and decorating the splendid tabernacle. This example shows clearly the collective wealth and egoism of the surviving patricians in an impoverished town.

It is understandable that such a mentality offended the common people, the shop workers. Their wretchedness and the memory of the plague only made their feverish souls more responsive to the communistic preaching of the apostles of poverty, the Fraticelli and the Spirituals (who were attached to the great Franciscan order).

The aggravation of social contrasts in the town, like the severe disequilibrium of the landed nobility, was a result of the plague. These effects of the plague intensified the hostility between the ruined nobility and peasantry (who refused to give up any of their newly won advantages) in the countryside, and between the rich bourgeoisie and the miserable proletariat in the cities. It was in this climate of class hatred brought on by the plague that there broke out, in the second half of the century, for different reasons, a series of violent social conflicts which had no equivalent in the preceding period. The rural insurrections included the Jacquerie (1358) and the Tuchins (1381–1382) in France and the Laborers (1381) in England. The insurrections of the urban proletariat included the Ciompi in Florence (1378), the Weavers in Gand (1379), the Harelle in Rouen (1380), and the Maillotins in Paris (1382).

Finally, the Black Death had a profound effect even on intellectual and spiritual matters. In striking the clergy severely, it brutally deprived the population of a large proportion of its spiritual guides; in depopulating especially the urban monasteries of the mendicant orders, it suddenly removed the intellectual elite among the clergy.

The vacancies so abruptly caused by the plague had to be filled. Everywhere new priests were quickly ordained and new monks tonsured. These were for the most part fairly young or fairly old people, neither group having any priestly experience or the moral and intellectual preparation needed to exercise the office worthily. Most of the new religious, as was true of certain of the surviving priests, were attracted to the priesthood only by benefices. They sought the most profitable ones, striving to accumulate several, and they worried little about the care of souls. During a crisis period when the population had the greatest need of its spiritual guides, worldliness, immorality, and ignorance suddenly developed among the clergy. Abandoned to themselves, often demoralized and panic-stricken, the people lived slack moral lives and their religion became little more than a collection of superstitions. Traditional practices, belief in liturgical prayers, the habit of common prayer, and in some places even the divine service disappeared. The pious turned to a more personal religion, while the more material satisfied themselves with superstition. Everywhere the emotional triumphed over the rational. Thus the stage was set for the criticisms of reformers, who, from the end of the century on, preached an inner religion based upon the Bible. These reformers had great sport deriding and making a scandal of the unworthiness of too many clerics.

The plague, which greatly aggravated the long-standing ill of unfit clerics, also hindered remedying it. The Order of Friars Preachers [the Dominicans] devoted itself to preaching and teaching, and constituted the intellectual elite among the clergy. The Black Death, as we have seen, depopulated the monasteries of the Order. Faced with either closing some monasteries and concentrating the survivors in others, or with replacing the deceased friars as quickly as possible to keep all the monasteries open, the superiors general chose the second solution. Now quantity was preferred to quality. A run to the monasteries began; the practice of offering ten- to fourteen-year-old children to the Friars Preachers as oblates became general.

Such recruits often lacked zeal or aptitude. Ignorance crept into Saint Thomas's order; the novices' studies were often insufficient, and the general meeting of 1376 emphasized that many young friars could neither read nor write. This grave intellectual decline did not allow the Dominican Order to rectify the new tendencies resulting from the deplorable recruitment of the clergy, itself also an effect of the shock of the Black Death.

The Black Death of 1348 caused general disorder throughout Europe. It is not astonishing that so violent an epidemic had such severe and lasting consequences. Actually the entire epidemic lasted at least a generation, and it was even longer before its demographic effects were wiped out. Both in violence and extent this was one of the most severe epidemics that mankind has undergone. Above all, the epidemic of 1348–1350 did not completely disappear. After the first great spate of killing, there followed during the next half-century sporadic outbreaks of the plague, which seems to have survived in a latent state almost everywhere. For example, there was the plague of 1361 in Aquitaine, the plague of 1362 in England (known as the second plague), the plague of 1363 in Florence and in southern France, the plagues of 1369 and 1375 in England, and those of 1371, 1374, 1390, and 1400 in Florence. These outbreaks once again showed the ineffectiveness of contemporary medicine and preventive measures. Throughout Europe they prolonged for several decades the effect of the 1348 epidemic.

Thus the Black Death of 1348, by the very violence of the blow it dealt mankind and by the magnitude of its consequences (reinforced by later outbreaks), clearly qualifies as a major historical event. It ended the prosperity which had prevailed in the West during the end of the thirteenth century and the first part of the fourteenth. It brought great misery everywhere and for a time impeded the course of political and military events. It promoted some profound social changes: the ruin of the nobility and the clergy, the rise of the bourgeoisie, the appearance of social strife between bourgeoisie and proletariat in the towns and between nobility and peasantry in the countryside. It also considerably hastened intellectual and moral change: the development of a lay spirit and the birth of national cultures. Finally, it caused, in an overexcited and restless population, the most frenzied and superstitious forms of religious life, which the decimated and substandard clergy could not correct. This is why certain historians, declaring how this universal event indeed ended a period, by oversimplification have wanted to see in the Black Death of 1348 the veritable terminus which separates medieval from modern civilization.

ÉLISABETH CARPENTIER, a member of the École
des Hautes Études in Paris, is concerned with late
medieval economic and social history. She has written
on several fourteenth-century subjects, including French
demography and a history of Orvieto and the plague
of 1348. This selection is drawn from an article
published in 1962 which remains the best survey in
recent historical literature concerning the Black Death.*

Élisabeth Carpentier

The Plague as a Recurrent Phenomenon

Epidemics have a history. For a particular region, or rather for a given continent, they spread during a longer or shorter period of time, then they lose their virulence and slowly or abruptly disappear, making room for new infections. It is readily admitted that the year 1348 was the true birth year in Europe of the Black Death, bubonic and pneumonic. This malady had certainly already reached Europe during the course of two previous large-scale epidemics: one in the fifth century B.C., immortalized by Thucydides, and the other during the reign of the emperor Justinian (A.D. 527–565). In addition several sources indicate that there were outbreaks of the plague during the Roman period and the early Middle Ages. But it was only in the fourteenth century that the plague became solidly entrenched in Europe; this fact alone justifies our study of the period. Speaking only in terms of the history of epidemics, we can say without exaggeration that modern Europe began in 1348.

At least two great "mortalities" occurred in the first half of the fourteenth century. The first, which struck a Europe already gripped by famine, ravaged especially the northern countries from 1315 to 1317. The second broke out in many places from 1340 to 1342, but was particularly violent in Italy. Modern scholars are given to conjecturing about these two

*From Élisabeth Carpentier, "Autour de la peste noire: famines et épidémies dans l'histoire du XIVe siècle," *Annales. Économies, Sociétés, Civilisations,* XVII (1962), 1080–1083. Translated by William M. Bowsky. Footnotes omitted.

epidemics, to which it is impossible to assign the name of a specific disease. According to the chroniclers, these "pestilences" in a few months killed a third or a fourth of the population in areas that were infected. Those who were killed were nearly always living under famine conditions and suffering from malnutrition. The contagious character of the disease is nowhere evident in the sources. According to the individual case the disease is spoken of as dysentery, cholera, typhus, or typhoid, etc. One thing does appear certain: these various maladies nearly always occurred under conditions of famine. The chroniclers' descriptions never contain any details that would allow us to identify these diseases with the plague. Thus in northern Europe, devastated by the famine of 1315, the people began to die of starvation. Afflicted with edemas and exhausted, they fell dead in the streets. It was only in the wake of this famine that an unidentified epidemic (described by some authors as a "violent infirmity") broke out.

The chroniclers change their tone when they speak of the Black Death of 1348. Whereas they had referred to previous epidemics by simply using the term mortality or pestilence, with regard to 1348 they judged it proper to give a detailed description of the new evil. Certain among them believed that it was the first manifestation of a universal disaster. Thus a chronicler of Orvieto declares that "The first universal plague broke out in 1348 and was the strongest." But to this he added the revealing enumeration: "second plague, 1363; third plague, 1374; fourth plague, 1383; fifth plague, 1389 . . ." A new writer completed the list with a "sixth plague, 1410." Others might have continued the list for the fifteenth century. These recurring outbreaks constituted a new, significant factor. Prior to 1348 medieval Europe had known numerous diseases (and even three severe epidemics), but all these had been isolated and due to particular, exceptional circumstances. At first the Black Death might have appeared similar to these, but contemporaries were quickly forced to face reality. They now had to endure a solidly entrenched, long-lasting illness that reappeared every ten to fifteen years with implacable stubbornness. This was the veritable drama that marked the entire late medieval period.

Without doubt it was a drama on the moral plane. The moral consequences of the Black Death of 1348 have been discussed extensively. Would it not be even more proper to speak of the moral impact of the recurring epidemics? It would be interesting to study in depth the consequences of the second epidemic, which created the awareness of a permanent evil. At Orvieto the reactions were symptomatic. Fear and panic appeared much more quickly than in 1348. Henceforth they would reappear at the least alarm. At the same time there developed a certain habituation to the presence of the plague.

Henri Dubled[1] notes that in Strassburg and Alsace "This series of huge 'mortalities' kept the people in a constant state of nervousness and fear." This twofold attitude—fear and a growing habituation to the plague—cannot but have deeply marked the mentality of the fourteenth and fifteenth centuries, but there has never been a study focusing on this particular aspect of the plague epoch.

The influence of recurrences of the plague on demographic, social, and economic evolution during the last

---

[1] Director of archives and museums of Carpentras, France, this scholar specializes in the history of Alsace and the Comtat Venaissin.—Ed.

centuries of the Middle Ages has been examined in recent years. Most authors who have studied the problem have come to the same conclusion: that the Black Death of 1348 produced vast human losses, but that these losses should have been rapidly made up, as were those of preceding mortalities. What was serious in the case of the plague was its systematic return, which decimated generation after generation, frustrating all attempts at demographic recovery. Josiah C. Russell's conclusions regarding the population of England[2] are most convincing. These are the human losses that he reported as resulting from each epidemic:

First epidemic (1348), 25 percent
Second epidemic (1360), 22.7 percent
Third epidemic (1369), 13.1 percent
Fourth epidemic (1375), 12.7 percent

It is normal that the mortality rate decreased from one epidemic to the next, because the malady lost its virulence at the same time that the immunity of the population increased. Nevertheless it is striking to see how closely the losses due to the second epidemic approached those of the first.

In order to understand better the consequences of the plague as well as the slow disappearance of these consequences, it is necessary on the one hand to emphasize that the effects of the epidemics were cumulative and on the other to consider the victims' ages. In this category Russell's study (using as a point of departure the privileged documents called the "Investigations after Death"), though criticized remains by far the most extensive made

to date. The plague of 1348 affected especially adults, particularly older men (this explains the high mortality rate among the ranks of the secular and regular clergy). As a result the younger generation was able to replenish the population. Unfortunately the second epidemic afflicted particularly children; this time the future was definitively compromised.

Russell's stress on the importance of the recurrence of the plague must not be limited to England. The idea has been applied to Provence by Édouard Baratier[3] and to the region of Toulouse by Philippe Wolff,[4] who states "As terrible as was the mortality of 1348, it is especially the repetition of the plague during the following decades that must have had the gravest consequences. . . ." For Germany . . . this idea was vigorously put forward in a distinguished article by Ernst Kelter.[5] On his part, Henri Dubled estimates that "the Black Death alone, would not have sufficed to cause such an acute and lasting fall in demographic potential." When the Black Death of 1348 and later outbreaks of the plague in the fourteenth and fifteenth centuries are considered in their entirety (rather than as isolated phenomena), as a permanent aspect of the later Middle Ages, one is inevitably confronted with the problem of the "depression" which characterized this period of plague.

---

[2] The author is referring to Josiah C. Russell's pioneer study, *British Medieval Population* (Albuquerque, N.M., 1948).—Ed.

[3] A specialist in the economic and social history of Provence.—Ed.

[4] A professor at the University of Toulouse and specialist in the economic and cultural history of southern France and Catalonia.—Ed.

[5] Author of a volume of governmental price regulation (Jena, 1935), Kelter in 1953 published a major article treating German economic life in the fourteenth and fifteenth centuries.—Ed.

EVGENII ALEKSEEVICH KOSMINSKII (1886–1959) headed both the department of medieval history at Moscow University and the medieval section of the Institute of History of the Academy of Sciences of the USSR. Kosminskii was granted full membership in the Academy of Sciences (1948), his nation's highest academic honor, and he probably is the Soviet historian of western European medieval history most highly regarded by his peers in the West. His *Studies in the Agrarian History of England in the Thirteenth Century* (1956) is a major scholarly contribution. In the following selection he debates with Western historians the periodization of the economic history of western Europe, and in particular whether the fourteenth and fifteenth centuries can be considered a period of economic decline.*

Evgenii Alekseevich Kosminskii

The Plague Deemphasized

It is necessary to acknowledge that the authors of the report to the Tenth [International] Congress [of Historical Sciences] approach the question of a new periodization for medieval economic history with great caution. They do not speak of "periods"; instead, they employ the term presently current in Western historiography: "long-term trends." This term, which has not yet been definitely adopted, designates a "phase of long duration" in economic development, a phase that is determined by a predominant, characteristic tendency, in essence a tendency to progress or to decline. These phases must be distinguished from fluctuations of short duration. This report treats the

phase of long-duration economic decline (or to speak with greater caution, of economic depression or stagnation) which characterized the European economy of the fourteenth and fifteenth centuries, more precisely from 1320 to 1330 until the last quarter of the fifteenth century. This century- or even century-and-a-half-long phase exists between two phases of progress as a "long-term trend."

In light of this theory the development of the European economy from the eleventh to the fifteenth century is presented as follows: the period from the eleventh century until the beginning of the fourteenth century is characterized as an epoch of economic progress despite some

*From Eugen A. Kosminsky, "Peut-on considérer le XIVe et le XVe siècles comme l'époque de la décadence européene?" in *Studi in onore di Armando Sapori,* vol. 1 (Milan: Istituto Editoriale Cisalpino, 1957), pp. 559–569. Translated by William M. Bowsky. Footnotes omitted.

traits of decline. There was vigorous population growth, extension of cultivated land, increase in agricultural and industrial production, technical progress, strengthening of internal and external commerce, and a rise in the prices of agricultural products.

The depression began from 1320–1330 (perhaps even earlier). Population began to decline (the epidemics of the fourteenth century are not considered the chief cause; they merely augmented a decline previously begun). Agricultural lands were partly abandoned, towns began to fall into decay, agricultural and industrial production diminished, technical progress was arrested, commerce was reduced (especially international commerce), and prices dropped. In the last quarter of the fifteenth century a new climb began, accompanied by a rise in prices. The depression developed gradually and was not catastrophic. It too disappeared gradually. This depression was not a disaster for the people of Europe; a considerable number of segments of the population were even able to ameliorate their economic condition during this epoch. While wage earners and peasants bettered their condition, the great landed proprietors suffered. . . .

The process of economic evolution in Europe during this epoch is extremely complex, and it is only by bringing together and evaluating contradictory facts that one can begin to form a general opinion of the "predominant tendency."

The chronological outline of the "depression" is not clear. Certain scholars put its beginning at the end of the thirteenth century (even in the middle of that century), while others prolong its duration until the beginning of the sixteenth century. The depression did not affect all the countries of Europe, and those affected did not all suffer equally. It manifested itself differently in different regions of each country and in different branches of the economy. Frequent local, partial recoveries of short duration occurred. Often the depression of former, traditional industrial and commercial centers was merely a result of the shift of such economic centers to new places, sometimes from the town to the countryside. The decline of one branch of industry was often compensated for by the development of another, as can be seen in places where cloths of great value were supplanted by cheaper cloths and by cotten and linen. Abandonment of former commercial highways was sometimes caused by a change to new means of transportation, more advantageous in respect to expenses, duties, etc.

Thus the decline or depression can only be viewed with substantial caution. The matter is still more complicated, since related questions are dealt with very unequally in the specialized literature and a problem must frequently be assessed in light of merely some conjectures or insufficient facts of a fortuitous nature.

Study of this problem in different countries can only reinforce the impression of uncertainty and raise the legitimate question of whether one can rightly speak of decline or even stagnation as the predominant tendency of the European economy in the fourteenth and fifteenth centuries. . . .

With regard to the countries of eastern Europe, it seems to me that the question of a decline in the "last centuries of the Middle Ages" is not even posed.

The situation in Germany is more complicated. The absence there of a unified national economy hinders the fixing of general developmental stages and the determination of their tendencies. The author (Paul Johansen) claims that the evolution of the economic regions of Germany was determined primarily by the rural economy, not by industry and commerce. In northern and eastern Germany, despite the partial abandonment of cultivated land *(Wüstungen)*, it is seen that grain production was sufficient to enable the Order[1] and the Hanse[2] to maintain a policy of exportation. One can suppose that the depression was not felt there. Johansen believes that certain symptoms, for example, the consequences of the Black Death, have often been exaggerated by scholars. In general, one can form an idea of the German economy in that epoch only be taking into account individual regions. Johansen grants that Germany too was affected by the depression, but in a different way from the countries of the west. The expansion of southern German towns was in contrast with the economic evolution of other regions. (Some investigators think this expansion should be put at a later date.) In sum, for Germany the question of depression has not been definitely resolved; it still requires a great deal of research.

Italy does not fit into the picture of general economic depression. In the second half of the fourteenth century a series of symptoms of depression was provoked by the Black Death, by the loss and displacement of certain markets, by wars, etc., but this did not constitute a general depression of economic activity. Italy quickly recovered its losses and the fifteenth century was an epoch of new economic expansion. The question of agricultural production and commerce

in grain has been posed, but hardly studied. In the textile industry we definitely see no decline. There was only a partial shift of industry into the countryside and a change to different fabrics; other branches of the textile industry (that is, silks) also developed here and there. In the fifteenth century there was verifiable progress in banking. Italian monetary capital stimulated economic progress in other countries, especially in the lands of the Iberian Peninsula.

We do not possess enough facts to speak of a decline or depression in another advanced area of Europe: the low countries. After studying this region, Charles Verlinden finds that the doctrine of a total depression of long duration (for this area) must be revised. He recognizes the lack of study on this whole question and indicates a series of phenomena which definitely do not correspond to the characteristics of a general depression. What appears as a decline was basically a shift in activity to another economic region, a shift into another branch, or, indeed, a market displacement. The decline of former economic centers was compensated for by the growth of new ones. Verlinden states that he would find it difficult to admit the possibility of a general depression on the eve of the greatest economic boom in the history of the low countries.

We are not sufficiently justified in speaking of a century-long depression in the states of the Iberian peninsula. Verlinden focuses his attention particularly on a tendency toward price decline, which is observed in the peninsula during the fifteenth century (in some areas earlier and in some later).

He finds the dominant cause of this decline in internal factors: population increase, the development of industry and commerce, and finally the gradual increase in the availability of precious

---

[1] This reference is to the Teutonic Knights, originally a crusading military order, later reconstituted and transferred to the German eastern frontiers.— Ed.

[2] The Hanseatic League, a powerful association of north German towns that existed primarily for trading purposes.— Ed.

metals. The economic fluctuations of this period were advantageous to those with salaries, but of very little advantage to those making a living from the land. But all these factors together are not sufficient as grounds for qualifying this epoch as one of depression.

Thus, characterization of the fourteenth and fifteenth centuries as a period of depression or even stagnation is dubious in regard to most European countries. In the final analysis, this characterization can only possibly be applied to two countries: France and England.

There is no doubt that a depression and decline occurred in France. But it must be remembered that no European country, except the Byzantine Empire, was as devastated as France in the fourteenth and fifteenth centuries. It is easy to see that the symptoms of the depression appeared most distinctly in the regions most stricken by the war. But even for France one must be careful in speaking of a depression at the end of the Middle Ages. Michel Mollat, after indicating the extreme diversity in price evolution, the confusion of the monetary system, the short-term fluctuations in the economy, varying greatly in different categories and regions, observes that "difficult times" began in France during the thirteenth century and that these difficulties manifested themselves in the phenomena of the decline and "recoveries" which succeeded each other, caused by different factors in the agrarian economy, in monetary circulation, and in the political situation. The general rise in all branches of economic life began only in the last decades of the fifteenth century. "At first diversity, then a general movement." It is in this that Mollat sees the mark of the passage from a compartmentalized and regionalized economy to an "open" economy.

Thus, it is difficult to speak of a depression, in terms of a total economic tendency of long duration, although symptoms of decline did exist. But is it not possible that these symptoms resulted principally from the political situation (the Hundred Years' War and internal conflicts)?

Finally there is England, which seems to be the classic example of the fourteenth- and fifteenth-century economic depression. It must be admitted that it is in England that most of the sources of medieval economic history have been preserved, that there are more detailed figures available for the history of prices and wages in England than elsewhere, and that the question of the economic depression has been studied there with the greatest care, especially by the eminent economic historian Michael M. Postan and his school. Nevertheless, the results still remain hypothetical and disputable.

But how do advocates of the theory of economic decline in fourteenth- and fifteenth-century Europe explain the causes of the decline?

The authors of the report recognize that the causes of the decline were many, but they still search for the fundamental cause. Political causes and wars, especially the Hundred Years' War, played a certain role, especially, for example, in the decline of maritime commerce. But the authors hesitate to place these among the fundamental causes of the general depression. They find too that attempts to attribute the depression to the drop in the price of agrarian products and the rise in the price of industrial products are not justified. The crisis in the international precious metals market also seems to them to be a rather unlikely explanation. The authors of the report, especially Postan, claim that the fundamental (but not sole) cause of the depression and its characteristic traits is a demographic factor: the decline in the population of Europe during this epoch. We said above that this decline is definitely not explained by the devastations caused by the great epidemics of the period. On the contrary, the devastating force of the fourteenth- and fifteenth-century epidemics resulted from the fact that they were unleashed on a population already affected by a decline. But if this is the case, how do we explain the decline? Postan offers a "Malthusian" explanation for the population drop. "Nature punishes man for having asked too much of her." The rapid population growth of the eleventh to the thirteenth century resulted in overpopulation, in "population pressure on the land" which caused the cultivation of marginal lands and the rise of food prices. Population grew faster than food supply; this caused a drop in living standards for most of the population. It also caused a halt in population growth and later its decline. All this was aggravated by the crises of the fourteenth century, by a series of famine years, by wars, and by the Black Death and the epidemics that followed it. The population decline can also explain such phenomena as the drop in wheat prices, the reduction of cultivated lands, the general diminution of agricultural products, the diminution in the volume of exports, the rise in wages, the decline in the revenues of the great landed proprietors, and at the same time the stability and even the partial amelioration of the living standards of a large part of the working population. The equilibrium between population size and means of existence, caused by the diminution of the population, led to a new economic rise and at the same time to a population increase in the last quarter of the fifteenth century.

All the same we must repeat that the authors, Professor Postan in particular, insist on the hypothetical character of their conclusions and on the need for further research on the subject.

We too are of the opinion that the question of whether one can qualify the fundamental tendency in fourteenth- and fifteenth-century European economic history as one of decline (or only stagnation) and the question of the real causes of the symptoms of the depression placed in this epoch can be clarified only by study of the sources themselves, research which at present has only begun. But at the same time we believe that it is necessary to pose simultaneously a number of general questions, necessary for determining the character of further research. My remarks have value only for this purpose.

I will focus my attention by preference on the economic "depression" in England, where the situation is the clearest and the best studied.

We must return to the question raised at the beginning: Can one study the symptoms of the economic depression without linking them to the historically determined mode of production that dominated the epoch, to changes in the distribution and character of landed property, and to class relations and class struggles? Would it not be possible to consider the so-called decline as really a progressive phenomenon; the decline of old institutions being compensated for by the growth of new ones?

If the question is approached from this point of view, the course of English economic life in the 14th and 15th centuries must be seen as progressive rather than otherwise. The regime of serfdom and forced labor collapsed. Money rents supplanted compulsory labor service; this and other factors caused a general lowering of feudal rents and a decline in peasant exploitation. The greatest part of the land became "free property," in the sense intended by Karl Marx in Volume I, Chapter 24, of *Capital.* Production for market became increasingly common among the peasantry; differentiation was accentuated; conditions became favorable for the development of capitalistic farming. The progressive role of the agrarian population became more and more pronounced; the peasants gradually secured markets for their agricultural products and struggled with perseverance against feudal exploitation. The fourteenth and fifteenth centuries are the classic age of great antifeudal uprisings, which despite their lack of success had a progressive character. Incidentally, the demands of the peasants during the revolt of 1381 were almost all realized in the fifteenth century.

Can one consider these processes a by-product of the population decline, which caused such phenomena as the drop in wheat prices and the rise in wages of agrarian workers, and place them within the general framework of the economic depression?

And can the decrease in population itself (hypotheses and conjectures still dominate the calculation of its dimensions and chronology) be explained without reference to the distribution of property and the predominant forms of exploitation? If population growth actually began to stop well before the Black Death (which itself resulted from the increasing misery), can this be explained only by overpopulation and "population pressure on the land," or can it be better explained by an intensification of feudal exploitation, which increasingly deprived the peasants of the greatest part of their production?

Can one speak of overpopulation in Europe at the end of the thirteenth century or even earlier? We doubt it. What especially raises doubts is the unusual population increase in the twelfth and thirteenth centuries.

It is difficult to determine the amount of population increase that occurred from the eleventh century to the beginning of the fourteenth, but it is even more difficult to determine how much the increase in cultivated land retarded population growth. The large number of small lots of land at the end of the thirteenth century is not adequate to account for an increase in human misery. The small lots, especially those of free tenants, were sometimes considerably augmented by pasturage rights; also the small tenants probably learned trades by which they earned additional income. In any case, it is very doubtful that the population of thirteenth-century Europe increased to such a point that the land suitable to be worked, cultivated, and colonized, no longer sufficed to nourish it.

The problem of rural poverty (and of poverty in general) becomes more real if we consider the amount of agrarian production absorbed by feudal rents. These rents, including the exactions of church and state, were constantly increasing. It must be noted too that on a great many thirteenth-century English manors there was an intensification of the most painful form of feudal exploitation, compulsory labor service. Finally the decrease in population in certain places (especially in regions where the system of servile-forced labor was most developed) can be linked to emigration to the towns, to less populated areas, and to centers of rural industry.

It follows then that the demographic factor (if it has really played the role attributed to it) cannot be examined without reference to the mode of production which dominated it.

We believe that the phenomena of depression, of which Professor Postan and the other scholars who share his viewpoint speak, cannot be studied apart from the subsequent course of the dominating feudal mode of production, which underwent a considerable crisis in a number of European countries during the fourteenth century. What was the nature of this crisis? M. Dobb and R. H. Hilton (whose explanation was not adopted by the authors of the article[3]) find that the feudal mode of production increasingly hindered the expansion of productive forces and that their expansion demanded the weakening of feudal exploitation. This weakening occurred at the end of the fourteenth and fifteenth centuries, in part under the influence of general economic causes (especially the competition of the peasant class) which rendered less advantageous the seigneurial economy based on the market, in part from peasant opposition which manifested itself in different ways—by poor work when at forced labor and by the great peasant uprisings. Feudal rent received by landed proprietors decreased. A considerable part of the land previously part of the seigneurial economy passed into the hands of the peasantry. We believe that there was no depopulation. Rather, the liquidation of the seigneurial economy, the commutation and diminution of feudal rent, which led to an amelioration of the peasant's situation and the expansion of simple commercial production, prepared a terrain suitable for capitalistic relations. A certain reduction in population (which would not be explicable without reference to the condi-

tions of development of the feudal system of production) could only aggravate and modify (not always equally) the march of this development.

But were there then indications of a decline? Yes, it seems so. The decline of the domanial economy—that is to say of gross agricultural production—the disasters caused by the Black Death and other epidemics, feudal anarchy, and the feudal wars during the growth of the great centralized monarchies were able to produce phenomena of depression.

Were these phenomena compensated for by rises in other spheres of economic activity? Could one suppose, for example, that the reduction of foreign markets was compensated for by the expansion of domestic markets? But it is difficult to determine if there was a balance, especially since our figures on the domestic market are not exact and those on the foreign market, which were formerly considered exact, have now been questioned.

Phenomena such as the decline of the gross feudal economy, caused largely by the market, the reduction of the ruling class's income, feudal anarchy, the decline of certain towns, and the decrease in population, seem to indicate a reduction, not an increase, in the domestic market. On the other hand, the increase in the income of certain (if not all) groups of the peasantry, the progress of industry in the countryside, the converting of almost all feudal rents to monetary form, the increase in state taxes (also in monetary form), all speak for the expansion of the domestic market.

It is perhaps necessary to pose another question first: Did productive forces decline during this epoch and did products increase or decrease in quantity? Certainly, if we calculate total quantity, there would be a decline if the population had decreased in number, but if we evaluate

---

[3] The article to which Kosminskii refers is the report to the Tenth International Congress of Historical Sciences. Rodney Howard Hilton is the author of numerous books and articles on medieval, especially English, economic and social history.

the amount of goods produced in relation to the number of people, there is no reason to suppose a decline. The majority of scholars believe, rather, that there was expansion. This is especially probable in the agrarian economy where the less productive work of the serf doing forced labor was replaced by that of the free peasant or the wage earner (whose wage had increased relatively).

During this age we see no technical progress in agriculture. Agrarian implements generally changed little during the Middle Ages. The principal role in the development of productive forces belonged not to tools, but to men, to their work habits, to work stimulants, and to the possibility of serving themselves. One can believe that these possibilities and stimulants must have increased in the economy of small, free producers. The organizational advantages introduced during the twelfth and thirteenth centuries in the great seigneurial economies were largely negated by the decline in productivity of forced labor.

One can admit that the quantity of wool produced in England diminished for a certain length of time and that the price of exported cloth did not fully compensate for the decline in the amount of wool exported. But although in the fifteenth century cloth exports, evaluated in monetary units, were less than wool exports in the fourteenth century, it was in the fourteenth and fifteenth centuries that the basis of the cloth export industry (which played such a great role in the development of English capitalism) was just being established. The decline of medieval towns is often explained by the shift of industry to new centers and by the beginning of a transformation of the local market into a national market.

Nevertheless, English society at the end of the fourteenth- and fifteenth-century "depression" differed greatly from the society that existed before this "depression." It was still a feudal society, but there were signs of the initial capitalist accumulation, conditions favorable for the development of capitalist relations in the industrial domain and the rural economy. We can conclude from this that, notwithstanding the phenomena of depression noted in the fourteenth and fifteenth centuries, these centuries, taken in their entirety, were not a period of general decline or even of stagnation in English economic evolution. Rather, this was a time in which decisive changes evolved, changes that moved England to first place in the process of European capitalist evolution.

The nature of the economy of the fourteenth and fifteenth centuries based only on English documents still cannot resolve questions which the fate of other European economies in this period suggest to us. A great deal of work remains to be done. But recent research, the results of which were presented at the tenth congress of historians, has cast doubt even on the theory of a European economic "depression" in the fourteenth and fifteenth centuries and would not permit the use of such a theory in laying the basis for a new periodization of the European economy.

I maintain the Marxist point of view which distinguishes in European history the succession of two fundamental socioeconomic formations: feudalism and capitalism. But it is necessary to discern in each of these formations some stages with some specific symptoms. We observe in the fourteenth and fifteenth centuries in certain European societies a stage that opens the way to the formation of capitalist conditions within feudal society, thus bringing about the decay of feudalism.

Study of the phenomena of "depression" which one notes in this epoch holds special interest for the Marxist historian; he must determine whether these phenomena are proper for a given stage in the evolution of feudalism or if they are only of specific and local character. It is then that we approach a more general question concerning "the costs," the inevitable phenomena of "depression" which precede and accompany all progress and which stand out with particular clarity at certain stages of a particular formation that has reached the summit of its evolution and is beginning to drop toward its decline. At any rate we do not believe that the study of problems of evolution and of "economic" decline is possible without examination of their relationship to the mode of production of the epoch, not forgetting that the succession of socioeconomic formations takes place in different countries at different epochs and in different ways.

A member of the Academy of Agriculture of France, the archivist and paleographer RAYMOND DELATOUCHE (b. 1906) has written on numerous aspects of late medieval French social and economic history. His work includes studies of western French feudal houses from the thirteenth to the sixteenth centuries and of medieval agriculture and population. The following selection is from a wide-ranging examination of the crisis of the fourteenth century in Western Europe.*

Raymond Delatouche

European Crisis:
The Plague or Moral Decline?

The crisis of the fourteenth century in western Europe has attracted the attention of historians for a long time. Following the expansion of the tenth through the twelfth centuries, and after the balanced blossoming of the thirteenth century, there opened a period of intellectual doubt, social strife, and economic contraction during which the characteristic traits of the Middle Ages disappeared and the first stirrings of the coming Renaissance dimly appeared.

In the search for causes, two major events stand out: the Great Plague of 1348–1350 and the Hundred Years' War, one fortuitous and the other the work of man.

Certainly the enormous, almost instantaneous loss of population caused by the plague and the lamentable situation that progressively enveloped France, until then the leading nation of western Europe, can be considered as the origin of a turning point in history. The sudden disappearance of half, in some places two-thirds, of the population, the decimation of elites, the sudden extinction of whole families, the transfer of property, the moral shock that resulted, all had a profound effect. And instead of a period of peace and calm in which the damage might have been repaired, there followed, particularly in France, a long chain of violence, destruction, and pillage. Even the church underwent great difficulties.

One is even more disposed to accord

*From Raymond Delatouche, "La crise du XIVe siècle en Europe occidentale," *Les Études Sociales,* n.s., no. 42–43 (1959), pp. 1–2, 4–6, 8–17, published by the Société d'Économie et de Science Sociales. Translated by William M. Bowsky. Footnotes omitted.

a fundamental importance to the Black Death when one realizes that the economy of the time was essentially based on agriculture, and agriculture on the work force. It is a fact that there was in the fourteenth century a distinct halt (in France at least) in agricultural progress; even worse, there was a noticeable regression. . . .

On examining the situation more closely, however, one perceives that the plague did not strike a completely healthy body, but a weakened organism which had been manifesting signs of trouble and disequilibrium for some decades. Historians, both local and general, economic and art historians, historians of thought, religious historians, rural and urban historians, population historians, and even genealogists have noticed, from the end of the thirteenth to the beginning of the fourteenth, signs of malaise, decline, and exhaustion.

Certainly, each of these scholars finds an explanation for this decline within the framework of his own research: local or regional conflicts, fiscal troubles, floods or droughts, plague or famine, the policies of central governments, the evolution of ideas, etc.

None of the explanations, however, completely accounts for the whole phenomenon, which, when seen in its entirety, gives the impression of a collective decline in vitality.

The crusades provide if not an image at least a striking symbol of the graphic curve in vitality from the eleventh to the thirteenth century. At the juncture of the eleventh and twelfth centuries there was a spreading wave of religious enthusiasm which aroused all Western Europe to attack the Muslims: a poor peoples' crusade, a barons' crusade, hosts of candidates for colonization—more than 200,000 (according to René Grousset's estimate) were massacred in

Asia Minor. In comparison the expeditions of Saint Louis seem thin streams that were lost without achieving their goals, the first in the sands of Egypt and the second only in Tunis.[1] At the end of the thirteenth century the last European settlements in Syria succumbed amid almost general indifference. From then until the nineteenth century Europe was on the defensive against Islam. . . .

Catastrophic theses do not hold up under examination. Certainly the linking together of rains or drought, scarcity, the weakening of physical resistance, plague, and depopulation appears logical. But even if these appeared exceptional to contemporaries, climatic or other such natural catastrophies are not peculiar to any given epoch. Only the Black Death of 1348, because of its extent, severity, and suddenness can be characterized as a decisive disaster. But the crisis manifested itself more than a half century before the Black Death struck.

One battle—to use war as an example —destroys a nation only if the defeat expresses in one notable event a profound decadence due to other than fortuitous causes. It is the same when a society succumbs in the face of transitory evils; the society must already have been ill. A natural catastrophe, moreover, can be a salutary stimulus, reawakening a society's energies, just as a military defeat can mark the beginning of a people's recovery.

The nineth and tenth centuries suffered from foreign invasion, devastation, and pillage much more than did the fourteenth century. Yet the tenth century saw the dawn of a civilization and the fourteenth its twilight.

If a natural cataclysm is clearly for-

---

[1] Louis IX of France (1226–1270) participated in the seventh and eighth crusades and died on the latter.—Ed.

tuitous, its destroying power often results from long negligence and lack of constraint. A flood may result from a storm, a winter of abnormal rains, but also from untimely deforestation or poorly maintained dikes. A famine may result from abnormal cold, but also from an absence of foresight, negligent cultivation, or a decline in commerce. Epidemics may result from unhealthy living, poorly maintained towns, stagnant ponds, and abandoned canals which cause swamps. Wars may result from the absence of political power, the loss of civic and military courage, indiscipline, lack of imagination, and internal weaknesses that arouse the envious ambitions of neighbors.

One cannot seriously believe that agriculture was no longer able to nourish a population supposedly grown too numerous. Certainly lands under cultivation at the end of the thirteenth century reached an extent that would hardly ever be surpassed. But so far as technology went, these lands were far from being exploited at the most intensive level conceivable. Even taking into account a lack of sufficient livestock, this last hypothesis [of overpopulation] remains questionable. The great importance of the production and export of wine proves that contemporaries were able to devote a large part of their land, labor, and fertilizer to luxury production. Furthermore, Édouard Perroy, who advanced the undernourishment theory, refutes it himself when he establishes that after the bad years of 1315 to 1317 there were better than average harvests and a drop in agricultural prices over a period of time, which is little compatible with a situation of endemic want.

If one advances an economic crisis as explanation for the medieval decline, one must first be sure, even now,

that economic crises are capable, in themselves, of causing the decline of a society; that is, that they are more than just epiphenomena, the manifestations of a more profound crisis. One should above all refrain from applying the contemporary notion of economic crisis to the thirteenth and fourteenth centuries. . . .

What is striking, from the end of the thirteenth century, is the collapse of moral potential, the loss of creative élan, the pursuit of leisure, even when leisure-time activities were of the highest quality—artistic, intellectual, and even religious. There are two words in the orison of the feast of the stigmata of Saint Francis of Assisi (the text of which may well date from 1337) which describe this decline well: *frigiscente mundo* (the world seems to grow cold).

When Saint Louis died on the Tunisian shore, a whole world view was dying with him. Sometimes he seemed a stranger even in his own milieu, often misunderstood even by members of his of his own entourage—by the faithful Joinville,[2] for example.

This decline in moral potential was accompanied by the growth of individualism, by the relaxation of social, religious, familial, feudal, rural, and urban bonds.

The decline in potential and the weakening of the creative spirit are especially perceptible in the ruling classes; the damage caused by this decline was greatest there too. The decline manifested itself on all planes; there are an infinite number of examples of it.

In the tenth and eleventh centuries the great ecclesiastical figures were the founders of monasteries, the builders. In the twelfth century a Saint Bernard

---

[2] Joinville (1224–1317) was the seneschal and longtime servant of Louis IX and wrote a *Life of Saint Louis.*—Ed.

took part in all the theological and philosophical controversies of his time —with God knows what vigor!—but at the same time he launched a crusade, intervened in international politics, and encouraged the spread of agrarian monasteries throughout Europe. These men of the tenth through the twelfth century believed that one could sanctify oneself by *creating* wealth. One risked peril when one was content simply to *enjoy* riches. In the thirteenth century this was clearly perceived by Saint Dominic and Saint Francis of Assisi, who energetically championed the virtues of poverty.

The old agrarian monastic orders became rentiers, deriving their income completely from the soil. The young mendicant orders quickly lost their conquering intellectual and religious ardor. Humbert de Romans, fifth superior general of the Dominicans, reproached his order for its lack of both missionary and scholarly zeal. There was a retreat from foreign evangelization, Greek was not studied, and this was one of the causes of the poor relations with the Byzantine Church.

There was no lack of candidates for canonical prebends, but a great many canons refused to enter higher orders and certain chapters could no longer maintain religious services.

The most extraordinary example of the moral decadence of the religious elite is furnished by the military orders. There were about 9000 chapter houses of the Knights Templars in Europe, but only a few hundred Templars took part in the last battles in Syria.

In the lay feudal world the military chief, the local chief of state, and the landed proprietor intent on maintaining his land gave way to the rentier and the royal functionary. The division of in-heritances, the devaluation of rents paid in silver coin, diminished the fortunes which were means of investment. The disappearance of the domanial regime in France separated the ruling class from the agriculturalists. The ruling class, living off the products of the land, became at the same time alienated from the land. The prevailing security diminished its military role. The advance of royal power reduced its role as the guardian of order. The taste for luxury multiplied its expenses. It tired of adventure and remained at home. Joinville himself refused to follow his master in 1270.

From an *arriviste,* the bourgeois merchant became a *parvenue.* In the earlier period the merchant had been fully occupied with his business, as had been his family. The great Italian businesses were family affairs, in which the family, including all of its possessions and activities, was involved without restriction. This family solidarity was the basis for the credit of the business. The merchant himself was usually on the road.

In the fourteenth century the merchant became sedentary. He was preoccupied with limiting his responsibility; he insured himself against risks by the purchase of lands, acquisition of rents, and the exercise of lucrative public functions. The lands purchased were not considered a new field of economic activity but an assurance of security.

The partnership was not only an appreciable technical advance. It had a moral aspect. As a partnership a business became an entity complete in itself, having its own life and autonomy, with which one collaborated in order to extract profit without completely engaging oneself and ones personal property in it.

Even the progress of culture, of the arts, contributed to diverting the wealthy from constructive activities and to the development of a taste for leisure among them.

The milieu of the universities did not escape this preoccupation with an established, comfortable situation. The universities tended to become more exclusive, multiplying their sources of revenue while increasing the rights from which they profited.

In the world of the artisan, it is notable that corporations do not seem to have been solidly established until the end of the fourteenth century. . . .

Corporations are seen by the historian, especially the legal historian, only through statutes regarding them, simple codifications of customs. The more complete and developed the statutes are, the more perfect the corporations seem. But this stage only arrives—the word arrives describes the matter well—at the moment when they have lost their dynamism, when they have become not only static, but, what one might call "stratifying."

This is indeed the picture that they present: "In large part," declares a French ordinance of 1348, "regulations [affecting corporations] are enacted more to favor and profit the persons of each trade, than for the common good." In this sense, one can say that the development of corporations in the fourteenth and especially the fifteenth century expresses the end of the vitality of the Middle Ages.

Parallel to this collapse of elites, a distension of social bonds manifested itself. The great crisis of the ninth and tenth centuries scarcely left in existence the Church, family, and domain, or the bonds of religion, blood, and land.

In the thirteenth century, familial ties became relaxed and narrowed. The decline in the birthrate seems to be the mark and maker of obsolescence. The

laudatio parentum, the authorization for alienations required from heirs of the same blood, a usage general in France from the ninth to the twelfth century, saw its sanction limited in the time before it fell into disuse. . . .

Feudal and domanial bonds: Serfdom declined in the face of massive enfranchisements; the obligations of the villain diminished. In the sharing of crops the share earned by work increased, that earned by capital diminished. The monetary commutation of military and agricultural obligations became common, and was even lightened because of monetary devaluation. The evolution of the feudal regime is clear: from the tenth to the twelfth century, feudal ties were strong at the base and loose at the summit; from the end of the twelfth century this situation was reversed—feudal ties became relaxed at the bottom and strengthened at the summit.

The bonds of urban and rural communities: These communities developed under the force of two necessities. It was necessary to group together in order to construct and administer new projects —to construct churches, charitable establishments, bridges, to establish markets and organize drainage and irrigation, and so forth. It was necessary to group together also for security and to regularize relations with the local lord. Usually the arrangement resulted from a realistic agreement between two powers equally sure of their rights, equally determined to have them respected. The decline of feudal power and security, and the weakening of creative capacity caused the disappearance of the salutary conditions which had been at the origins of the communal movement. So paralleling the feudal decline was a decline of communal associations.

Religious bonds: Parochial bonds

which rivaled the groupings encouraged by the mendicant orders and bonds even within the interiors of some traditional monasteries. A series of cartulary texts demonstrates the economic crisis which struck landed proprietors from the end of the twelfth century. Most curious is the remedy employed by religious houses against this crisis. A piece of land or a priory especially much in debt was detached and assigned to an individual monk who was detached from the monastery to manage it, sometimes with the aid of his family. During the same epoch the goods of certain chapters, Mans for example, were divided into individual prebends in order to improve their administration. The Cistercians relaxed their early rule, and no longer recruited lay brothers, which represented a flight from humble manual labor. Papal expenses multiplied. "From a religious body with a common life," wrote Dom David Knowles[3] of the situation in England during the fourteenth century, one passes "to a college of clerics or to a chapter of resident regular canons."

Individualism manifested itself everywhere. It is clearly apparent in the liturgy. . . . The beginning of the thirteenth century marks a turning point in the evolution of liturgy. Individual prayer tended to replace communal worship.

The growth of individualism assumes a fundamental importance in agriculture. Individualism is repugnant to agriculture. The isolated individual is of little weight in agriculture, which demands long-term and large-scale planning, perseverance across centuries, courage, support, and, even more important, close

family ties. Agrarian production is delicately balanced and complex. It cannot with impunity be submitted to the hazards of successive division among heirs, of temporary ownership, and to the sole imperative of immediate profit.

Agriculture is not an isolated microcosm. The development of a given region reacts upon the development of others by example, work atmosphere, and techniques employed. Equally, all regions suffer from negligence in one. Livestock do not know the limits of fields, only of solid enclosures. Poor strains of grain and parasites are even more mobile. The smaller an area of agricultural production, the greater is its solidarity and the more numerous are the occasions on which that solidarity has to manifest itself so as to compensate for individual weakness, and the more necessary is the presence of an elite to promote effort and progress. The active cohesion of a rural community can be assured by a vigilant master or by an elite formed from among the administration of collective institutions. In all ways, it demands that men join character to intelligence. Without this elite, imposed or accepted, the rural community becomes a pillory, the framework of stagnation and mediocrity.

Only then does the growth of individualism become necessary, so as to burst the iron collar of the pillory. The poison becomes the medicine. It permits a new elite to show the masses new ways, to bring them into its following by persuasion, example, and eventually by diverse forms of constraint.

In the fourteenth century we are at the first phase of destructive egoism, that of individualism. Juridical institutions reconciling order and liberty, initiative and constraint, that had allowed prodigious earlier expansion in an atmosphere of work, now changed their

---

[3] Professor emeritus of Cambridge University and a Benedictine, Dom Knowles is one of the most eminent historians of medieval religion, particularly in England.—Ed.

meaning in the general atmosphere of noninterference.

The power of monopoly assured the most essential collective investments (mills, bakeries, etc.), the indispensable discipline of neighboring agriculturalists (harvest monopoly, etc.), but it constrained technical progress (by monopolies on grape vintage and on bulls and other reproducers, etc.). It gave a dismal cast to financial matters.

The division of property rights and real rights among many holders favored the multiplication of free hearths, productive credit, and constructive labor, whose fruit remained at least in part in the hands of the laborer; at the same time it protected the stability of development.

This now resulted in the pulverization of the land; it became burdened beyond measure by a veritable parasitism. For Normandy, Lucien Musset rightly notes, "Nothing is more manifest when one peruses the Norman cartularies. One sees in them an incredible pullulation of rent sales. Nearly all social classes took part in these alienations, even the most humble. This multiplication was so great that one can speak of a true division of land revenue between the rural farmer and the investor (usually a stranger to the actual work on the land), in general an ecclesiastic or a member or the urban middle class." The establishment of rents that were not balanced by an increase in productivity mortgaged the future for gain in the present. Short-term leases, when candidates for exploitation were numerous and active, restored the generative pressure of industry; but in France such leases appeared only sporadically, and candidates for exploitation were neither numerous nor active.

This society which had been lulled into a sense of security, lost the power of invention, of renewal. Not that inventive creativity is a social ability. Inventiveness is an individual faculty, and all centuries have their contingents of inventors. What is eminently social is the ability to adopt, utilize, and expand inventions; to make them yield their fruits.

The tenth through the twelfth centuries were exceptionally fruitful: in agriculture, for example, there was the horse harness; in navigation, the sternpost rudder; in industry, the water wheel and windmill; in architecture, first the Romanesque and then the Gothic style; in music, etc. In most cases it was not a matter of actual new discovery, but of importation, adaption, and generalization.

From the end of the thirteenth century, technical innovation ceased. R. H. Hilton correctly points out the similarity between this period and the Late Roman Empire. The armies of the late Empire were defeated by the barbarians because they failed to adopt the tactics and weapons of the barbarians. Similarly, in the fourteenth century the French army remained stubbornly attached to out-of-date tactics and weapons, insensible to the lessons it received or the misfortunes that followed it. It cherished the courage of the individual warrior, but it had lost intelligent flexibility and the sense of collective action.

Architecture remained stubbornly unchanging, keeping to its own well-worn rut. The flamboyant Gothic architecture reached a dead end in the waning thirteenth century. . . .

Rural architecture, too, exhibited this ossification. Heavy constructions of stone replaced those of wood, which had been light, inexpensive, and when necessary transportable. Stone constructions were a poor investment, as they were more costly than wood and made a person less mobile than did wooden ones. They were a factor of conservatism—a person was henceforth attached to his house and no longer able to take up his goods and emigrate—an obstacle to expansion and profitable change.

Among intellectuals inspirational sources did not dry up. In England, in particular, the movement that would give birth to empirical and experimental science took shape. But the forces of conservatism and habit were more powerful. They masked their rejection of innovation under a sterile care for perfection and absolute exactitude. . . .

The decline of elites, the relaxation of organic social ties, immobility, and stagnation evoked, particularly in France, what was described after World War I as a wave of indolence. Through one of those chain reactions which characterize social movements these consequences, became in turn evolutionary factors, and developed in two directions: administrative centralization and social conflict.

Central authority, bureaucratic administration, occupied the place vacated by powerless or dispossessed local authorities; it filled the vacuum left by the relaxation of organic social bonds, spontaneous or artificial. The resurgence of central government was a necessary reaction against anarchy. But in France and in the Church at least, the balance between the needs of order and of life, in appearance contradictory, in reality complementary, did not last long. Saint Louis preserved before his eyes, wrote Louis de Lagger, the ideal of a feudal monarchy that respected ancient acquired autonomies, according to Louis's motto of *Suum cuique* (to each his own). His functionaries were not so liberal. This class, which produced the jurists of Philip

the Fair, was full of men avid for power. Wherever and however they could, they worked to expand the administrative sector of the state. They found an excellent tool for this in Roman law, the law of the Late Empire, a period when society was in a state of decomposition and held together by a straitjacket of state controls. They now had an administrative science, the science of law. The members of this bureaucratic community, of similar background and aspiration, harmonized their actions around the power whose agents they were, just as in a modern technocracy. In advancing their designs, they profited from all the deficiencies of the local powers as well as from their anarchic attempts at reaction.

The administrative machine of Philip the Fair is a good example. Without awaking suspicion, it was able to stifle the powerful Templars[4] simultaneously throughout the kingdom. A score of years later, it executed for the monarchy the only precise census before the modern era.

For its part, the Roman Curia remedied the relaxation of voluntary discipline, profiting from it to develop a centralized administration.

These administrative machines were expensive, and they grew even more costly because of their natural tendency to proliferate. Mercenaries replaced personal military service. The feudal lords saw their revenues dwindle at the same time that their expenses grew. A resemblance to the Late Roman Empire becomes apparent in monetary artifices and in the strong grip of the fisc on the

---

[4] By the time of their destruction in France by Philip IV (1285–1314), the Templars—originally a crusading military order—had become a major banking institution and the object of suspicion because of their secret rites.—Ed.

taxable economy, which when it was not exhausted, remained stagnant. The fisc curbed inventiveness and movement in the economy.

This fixed society offered a choice terrain for social ills. . . . The services that the traditional elites rendered no longer compensated for the privileges they received. They scarcely continued to provide security—when they did perform their military function, they performed it badly—and their former administrative functions now fell to the central government or to local communities. In France they abandoned their traditional economic role. They no longer engaged in an exchange of reciprocal services with the people; they now appeared as parasites and aroused envy. The rift between the French nobility and people became tragically clear in the first battles of the Hundred Years' War. . . .

Speaking in absolute terms, it is probable that the general standard of living did not decline at the beginning of the fourteenth century. But in this motionless society no creative spirit arose to polarize ambitions. The *beati possidentes* (the well-to-do) became an exclusive class, stiffling the hope of others to rise. Men no longer came together to build; but they united to make claims. . . .

To conclude, this fourteenth-century crisis occurred especially in France, but France, by reason of its location, population, wealth, and previous role, held a preponderant place in Europe. Whatever affected France had profound repercussions everywhere. This crisis was a manifestation of the universal law of action and reaction; the price of too great an effort, too great a success; the price of the well-being and creativity of the

high Middle Ages. It was a price that was just as heavy as the earlier success had been complete. The natural advantages, the shock, after the Albigensian crusade,[5] of "communal" influences of Midi society, less appropriate for shaping the spirit during a period of decline, increased the lowering of potentiality that is quite natural after great creative epochs. The harsh ordeals of the fourteenth and fifteenth centuries, the liquidation of accumulated obstacles, the crushing of the population, and the commanding necessity of reconstruction which these entailed were necessary to reforge new outlooks and open new horizons for human development.

This simple thesis does not have the perfect unity which satisfies the modern spirit of the economic theorist. Rather, it appeals to disparate elements, sometimes far removed from one another in time. The eclipse of a society is not a sudden, simple phenomenon. For a long time fissures spread insidiously before cracks appear. In the same manner, violent collapses precede renaissances by many years.

The ideas developed above will appear strange to those who think that the Middle Ages was a period constantly menaced by famine, the scene of a continual struggle for survival. However these ideas would not be strange to contemporary medieval witnesses. . . .

The explanation we have presented will seem wholly obsolete, moralizing, indeed, in a word, "traditional." This is all the more reason to favor it.

---

[5] A crusade undertaken in the early thirteenth century against Cathar, or Albigensian dualist "heretics," who were particularly powerful and numerous in southern France.—Ed.

A fellow of the British Academy, MICHAEL M. POSTAN (b. 1899) is the doyen of economic historians of medieval England. He was a lecturer at the London School of Economics before becoming a professor of economic history and fellow of Peterhouse, Cambridge University. His many studies of industry, trade, agriculture, and population are based upon careful analyses of original sources and attempt to arrive at historically valid statistical patterns. The following is an excerpt from a survey of medieval economic history that he presented to the Ninth International Congress of Historical Sciences in Paris in 1950.*

Michael M. Postan

Malthusian Pressure and Population Decline

On broad and largely theoretical grounds a rise and fall in population would be compatible with all the phenomena which our evidence exhibits and should raise none of the objections to which other general explanations are open. When population rose agriculture expanded under conditions which economists would recognize as those of steeply diminishing returns, and agricultural prices were bound to rise. On the other hand, when population fell supplies of agricultural products would be more plentiful, relative to the amount of resources engaged in their production and relative to the demand for food, and prices would be correspondingly lower.

A rise and fall in population would also have a so-to-speak selective effect on prices in that they would produce a corresponding movement in the prices of agriculture products, but would have little effect on prices of commodities not greatly subject to diminishing returns, i.e. most industrial products.

All this is theory, and, like all theories, it may at first sight appear too simple to fit the infinite variety of medieval experiences; but it so happens that this particular argument also fits with what from independent evidence we have now learned about medieval population. The main trends of medieval population and the direct evidence available for their

*From M. M. Postan, "Histoire Économique. Moyen Age," in *IXe Congrès international des sciences historiques. Paris, 28 aôut–3 septembre 1950.* I. *Rapports* (Paris: Librairie Armand Colin, 1950), pp. 232–236. Footnotes omitted.

study will form a subject of a separate paper. One class of such evidence—that of occupation of the land—must however be dealt with here in greater detail. It is perhaps too far removed from the conventional interest of demographers and sufficiently wide in its implications as to touch on almost all the aspects of economic history covered by this paper.

For the earlier centuries of the middle ages the facts of internal colonisation, of new villages, and of new settlements provides our main evidence of rising population. In England, where the study of settlement is still in an embryonic condition, some light on the growth of population between the eleventh and the fourteenth century is thrown by manorial surveys. But in France and Germany, where the study of settlement has been more advanced and surveys are few, the evidence of internal colonisation has been rightly used as proof of growing numbers of men and women. *Mutatis mutandis* evidence of falling numbers in the later middle ages has been found in the abandoned holdings and in the contracting areas under cultivation. In this way the story of expanding and contracting population merges into that of expanding and contracting agriculture: which is as it should be in a society where agriculture was so important and was so predominantly "peasant."

Thus, prices, population and agricultural production reveal themselves as different aspects of the same process, going through more or less the same phases of development, combining and interacting in every important event of medieval economic history. But their very interaction makes it difficult to single any of them out as the prime mover of economic change. In some ways the movement of population was more fundamental than any of the other economic changes; yet it would be difficult to treat the population trends as the sole or final cause. The search for final causes, here as in other fields of history, will inevitably result in a circular argument. For if the fall and rise in population caused the general fluctuations of medieval economy, what caused the fall and rise in population? It is theoretically possible, but on historical grounds not very probable, that a biological factor was at work: some sudden mutation in the human capacity for procreation. The Black Death could perhaps be regarded as a biological catastrophe; yet it is doubtful whether the Black Death, even if taken in conjunction with other great epidemics of the fourteenth century, could by itself account for the population trend of the later middle ages. For one thing, signs of falling trends appear before the Black Death and do not disappear after the direct effects of the great pestilences should no longer have been felt. Of other more fundamental biological changes we know nothing, and I doubt whether anything about them worth knowing will ever be discovered.

Could the change be accounted for by geographical, above all climatic causes? There is every reason for thinking that the agricultural depression was ushered in during the second decade of the fourteenth century by a succession of disastrous harvests. In England a sequence of wet years and inundations spread ruin and famine over the countryside; in Germany and France the period between 1309 and 1323 was also punctuated by years of hard weather and low harvests. Some Scandinavian students have also blamed a climatic revolution for the permanent change in agriculture economics of West Norway and Iceland. Whereas both countries had been able to supply their own bread before the four-teenth century, they became greatly de-pendent on imports in the late middle ages, and to all intents and purposes ceased to grow their own corn.

The argument is plausible but inconclu-sive. As far as England goes, one or two decades of bad crops would not account for an economic trend lasting a century and a half. Even if it were proved that during that time the eastern coastline of England sank and a permanent change occurred in the hydrography of Britain, it still remains difficult to understand why climatic changes which were suffi-ciently "permanent" to depress English agriculture until the last quarter of the fifteenth century, should yet have allowed an agricultural boom in the sixteenth century. As for West Norway and Iceland, it still remains to be proved that they had been able to support themselves out of their own food production in the ear-lier centuries, and that the decline of arable farming in the later cen-turies was not due to purely economic causes, such as the influx of cheap grain from the Baltic.

We are thus inevitably thrown back upon the more conventional and more purely social explanations. By analogy with other and similar ages in European history or with other civilisations simi-larly conditioned, historians and econo-mists will inevitably think of the inherent tendencies of populations on the Mal-thusian level of existence. Our knowledge of the demographic trends in the over-populated countries of the Far East, but above all recent studies of the Swedish population in the seventeenth and eigh-teenth centuries and of the Irish popula-tion on the eve of the potato famine, give us some insight as to what might happen to over-populated countries on a margin of subsistence. In Ireland the potato, which had borne well on newly-reclaimed land, suddenly gave out in the late forties mainly through plant disease; and popu-lation, which had previously added to its potato crops as it married and bred, sud-denly found itself faced with famine. It will not be too fanciful to project a some-what similar story into the facts of the middle ages and to see in the falling production of the later centuries a natural punishment for earlier over-expansion. As long as the colonization movement went forward and new lands were taken up, the crops from virgin lands encour-aged men to establish new families and settlements. But after a time the marginal character of marginal lands was bound to assert itself, and the honeymoon of high yields was succeeded by long periods of reckoning, when the poorer lands, no longer new, punished the men who tilled them with failing crops and with murrain of sheep and cattle. In these conditions a fortuitous combination of adverse events, such as the succession of bad seasons in the second decade of the fourteenth cen-tury, was sufficient to reverse the entire trend of agricultural production and to send the population figures tumbling down. The Black Death and the other great epidemics of the second half of the fourteenth century decimated the popula-tion of villages and towns, but the reasons why the recovery was slow and fitful may well have been that the epidemics oc-curred at a time when population and production were in any case moving downward.

This hypothesis is tentative in the extreme; a mere guess which may well turn out to be untrue. It is suggested here not in order to account for the popu-lation trends but in order to underline the complexity of historical causation. The growth and decline of population was probably the most fundamental of all the processes behind the increasing and declining production; yet it may itself have been influenced by upward and downward trends in medieval agriculture. Further study may reveal other forces behind the population movement—above all forces springing from revolutionary and irreversible changes in constitution of the family in time of agricultural expansion.

DAVID HERLIHY (b. 1930), professor of history at the University of Wisconsin and one of the most innovative of the current generation of American scholars, is a specialist in medieval and early Renaissance economic and social history. His published works, which include *Pisa in the Early Renaissance* (1957), suggest new approaches that may yield valuable historical information from the extant meager source materials. The following pages are a stimulating example of his work.*

David Herlihy

Malthus Denied

The more we learn of European populations before the plague, the more we must be amazed at the extraordinary numbers of people the medieval community had come to support.

Pistoia's population is no exception. At about 1244, the entire countryside of Pistoia was maintaining . . . about 34,000 persons settled within an area of about 900 square kilometers. This represents a density of rural settlement of about 38 persons per square kilometer. The total population of medieval Pistoia, including approximately 11,000 then residents of the city, would be about 45,000, which means a density of settlement of about 50 persons per square kilometer. This remarkable density was achieved, it must be added, even before 1250 and within a contado where over one half the land was comprised of high and inhospitable mountains.

Tuscany's more favored towns and more fertile territories in the thirteenth century were even more densely settled, not to say glutted. . . .

It is instructive to consider the implications of population densities which, even before 1250, reached and surpassed 50 persons per square kilometer. If all Tuscany shared the same density of population that Pistoia had attained by 1244— and since fully one half the Pistoiese contado was thinly settled high hills and mountains, that is not unlikely—the Tuscan province would have contained an astounding 1,200,000 persons even before 1250. Not until well into the nine-

*From David Herlihy, *Medieval and Renaissance Pistoia* (New Haven, Conn.: Yale University Press, 1967). Copyright © 1967 by Yale University. Pp. 112–120. Footnotes omitted.

teenth century would Tuscany again attain that figure. According to E. Fiumi's[1] not unreasonable estimate, the Tuscan medieval population at its height was "not less than" two million people.

With a relatively low level of technology and inefficient transport, how could the medieval economy have fed and employed such enormous numbers? Only at the cost, it would appear, of forcing thousands and tens-of-thousands to eke out their living on the bare margin of subsistence. In 1302, a year of scarcity, the commune of Siena undertook a public distribution of food, and the poor and indigent were found to number 15,000.

The Florentine chronicler Giovanni Villani was himself shocked to surmise that in 1330 the paupers of the city of Florence seemed to surpass 17,000. And poverty in the countryside was undoubtedly more gripping, if less conspicuous.

Poverty in turn brought poor nutrition, weakened physical stamina, and induced high susceptibility to disease. There can be little doubt that the great mortalities of the plague were closely linked to the poor nutrition and bad health of substantial numbers of the population. Many of the great plagues seem to have had the way prepared for them by famine and scarcity in the preceding years. The epidemic of 1340, first of the really great recorded killers, followed hard upon a year of want in 1339; two years of scarcity preceded the Black Death of 1348. And death from the plague followed dearth again in 1388–89.

A huge population, massive poverty, endemic malnutrition, shocking mortalities and a catastrophic population decline—these are unquestionable facts, and the Malthusian diagnosis of the

late-medieval crisis finds order and relationship among them. Does the fourteenth-century population plunge indeed present for us a true historical example of a classical Malthusian crisis?

Here, however, some reservation must be expressed. It is one thing to recognize the existence of a precarious balance between population and resources on the eve of the Black Death, and quite another thing to attribute the behavior of the demographic curve primarily to the impact of plague and famine upon an excessively swollen population. Rather, a careful examination of our data gives several substantial reasons for doubting that the shape of the curve does indeed follow the lines to be expected from an exclusively Malthusian diagnosis.

There is, to begin with, the pace and pattern of the population decline. The high mortalities of 1348 may with great plausibility be explained by malnutrition and by the inordinate numbers of consumers which induced it. But if Pistoia was overpopulated in 1344, was it still overpopulated in 1392, when the population was less than one half its former size? Yet its population continued to fall, well beyond the point where one may continue to speak of inadequate resources.

There is this further and, I think, decisive fact for rejecting an exclusively Malthusian interpretation for the depopulations of the fourteenth century. The plague of 1348 did not strike against a population blindly seeking to increase. The population had been stable or even declining at Pistoia for a century before the Black Death. The rural population of 1344, four years before the plague, had already shrunk by 23 per cent from what it had been one hundred years earlier. Moreover, for other Tuscan areas there are indications that the rural population was stagnant or declining well before the

---

[1] Enrico Fiumi is one of the outstanding scholars in the field of Italian medieval economic and social history. — Ed.

Black Death. At San Gimignano, the density of rural settlement had apparently reached its height by 1290 and by 1332 had already diminished. It is more difficult to judge population movements in the Florentine countryside, for which surveys for only a few scattered rural communes have survived. But such surveys still convey the strong impression that rural population was stable or even declining for at least a half-century before the Black Death.

The great demographic crash of the fourteenth century was not triggered by nor was it a direct reaction against a population expanding too rapidly. If population size alone were the nemesis of the medieval community, it would be hard to understand why the Malthusian reckoning had not occurred in the middle thirteenth, rather than the middle fourteenth century.

Perhaps the chief weakness and omission of a purely Malthusian diagnosis of the fourteenth-century population collapse is its failure to recognize the importance of birth rates. It assumes that these rates were high and constant, and that the population would automatically and mechanically have continued to grow until its very size would have called down upon itself violent checks and readjustments. The picture in fact is more complicated. Our own consideration of the Catasto of 1427[2] has shown that birth rates were not at all fixed and stable, but were highly sensitive to a variety of influences. It is, moreover, a recognized demographic fact that even apparently small fluctuations in births can have profound effects on the direction and degree of population changes. No analysis of the great depopulations of the late Middle Ages can be complete without attention

paid to the elusive but perhaps critical factor of births. . . .

We have two rough but useful indications of reproductive patterns in the thirteenth and fourteenth centuries: the long-term movement of the population and the apparent size of households.

The thirteenth century was comparatively free of major external checks upon population expansion. But even in the century's early decades demographic growth had weakened, ended or was already reversed. The birth rate in this epoch could have been only high enough to maintain the size of the community, and did not accomplish even that too successfully.

The plagues of the fourteenth century were terrible in their carnage, but they alone do not explain the failure of the population to rebound from them, as, in later periods, under more favorable circumstances, it was clearly able to do. Thus, in spite of plagues in 1416 and 1418, and another in 1423 which allegedly left the city deserted, the urban population actually increased between 1415 and 1427 by 20 per cent. This must mean that the birth rate reacted quickly and effectively to the challenge of losses, and the population in 1427, with an astounding fertility ratio[3] of 1170, shows the levels to which it could rise. So also, the losses due to the plague of 1400 are well-documented: one half the population in the city, and the same in the countryside. But even here, for all the dimensions of its losses, the population was able to make a quick recovery. The rural population was 11,364 in 1391; in 1401, only one year

---

[2] A census of the Florentine state, including Pistoia, compiled to provide a basis for taxation.—Ed.

[3] "This shows the ratio of children aged 0 to 4 years in the population to women of child-bearing age, usually taken as 15 to 44. At Pistoia in 1427, children so defined numbered 3364 and women 2877. This gives the . . . fertility ratio of 1170 (or 1.17 children per woman." Herlihy, *Medieval and Renaissance Pistoia*, p. 93,—Ed.

after the plague which carried off half its numbers, it was 10,027, almost regaining its former size.

The fourteenth-century population, on the other hand, showed no comparable power to make good its losses. The failure of the birth rate to respond to the stimulus of deaths, more even than the deaths themselves, seems the root cause of the shocking population plunge of the fourteenth century.

More evidence of a comparatively low reproductive rate even in the thirteenth century comes from the apparent size of households in the Book of Hearths.

The Book, to be sure, records only the names of heads of households, not the number of persons they contained. However, the names themselves give indirect evidence concerning household size. Where women appear in large numbers at the head of households, the average size of the homes must be small, as some women were not marrying or remarrying and many widows were not living with their married children. In 1427, for example, out of Pistoia's 2507 rural households, 191, or 7.6 per cent, were headed by a woman, and this corresponds to a household size of 4.65 persons. In the city, on the other hand, where the number of homes headed by women was substantially larger (264 out of 1247, or 21.1 per cent), average household size was correspondingly smaller, only 3.6 persons.

In the Book of Hearths of ca. 1244, the number of women appearing as household heads is high, approximately 714 out of 7312, or 9.8 per cent. This figure, it must be noted, cannot be considered exact; the sex of many of the persons listed in the Book cannot be certainly established through their names alone. And of course, upon this rough figure it would be impossible to base a precise estimate of average household size. But this high percentage of women at the head of hearths does show that the homes of ca. 1244 tended to be small, and probably could not have counted more than the 4.65 persons which they averaged in 1427. This was a small household in 1427 (the plague, after all, had struck only three years before, and the population was still in the process of recovering). It was also a small household in the thirteenth century.

The Book of Hearths shows further that in ca. 1244, as in 1427, the size of households, and presumably the birth rate, was affected by the social and economic status of their members. While the Book of Hearths gives no direct indication of a household's wealth, it does distinguish the homes of nobles from those of commoners. Noble households, which may be presumed to be the wealthier, appear also to have been the larger. Of noble hearths, 6.5 per cent were headed by a woman (17 out of 262), well below the 9.8 per cent representative of the entire community. The wealthy, even in the middle thirteenth century, were supporting larger households and presumably more children than the disadvantaged poor. One of Pistoia's noble and wealthy families, the Cancellieri, was so prolific as to attract the comment of chroniclers. Appearing only in the early thirteenth century, it could boast, in three generations, of more than 100 men of arms.

We are not without contemporary comment stressing the critical importance of births in the growth and decline of the population. In 1425, St. Bernardino attributed the dwindling numbers of Siena and Milan specifically to the failure of many young people to marry, and implicitly to the low birth rate which their reluctance engendered. Leon Battista Alberti,[4] in his *Libri della famiglia*, de-

---

[4] An Italian architect and humanist (1404–1472). —Ed.

voted a long section on how to make the family "populous." He noted the problem of young men who refrained from marriage "because of poverty." He urged their older and richer relatives not only to encourage them with exhortation and example, but also to donate to them a "suitable sum" for their needs, "as if to purchase the growth of the family." Otherwise, the family would fall in numbers and wealth, and perhaps disappear entirely, as many had.

These then seem to be the relative roles of plagues and famines, of overpopulation and of births in Pistoia's late medieval population history. The plagues, for which famines often enough prepared the way, took a fearsome toll, and mortalities from them were certainly heightened by poor nutrition stemming from overpopulation. The demographic plunge of the fourteenth century cannot, however, be taken as an example of a classical Malthusian crisis. A precarious balance between population and resources seems a fact of Tuscan rural life for as far back in the thirteenth century as our sources permit us to discern. The importance of overpopulation was probably greater in worsening social and economic conditions, and thus adversely influencing the birth rate, rather than as a direct provocation of plague and famine.

Although natural disasters clearly played a role of major importance in Pistoia's demographic history, their impact was apparently aggravated, and recovery from them delayed, by a low and unresponsive birth rate. The birth rate was in turn very sensitive to the social conditions under which Pistoia's families were living. In 1427, and undoubtedly too in the thirteenth century, poor people were having difficulty supporting children and maintaining their numbers. The willingness or ability of Pistoia's society to reproduce was strongly influenced by the extent and degree of poverty within it.

The evidence, scanty though it is, still suggests that bad and deteriorating social conditions under which numerous Pistoiesi had come to live by the late thirteenth century played a major role in halting the demographic expansion of the Middle Ages, and in worsening and prolonging the great depopulations of the fourteenth century. Conversely, the renewed if modest population growth of the fifteenth century implies that the conditions of life were then improving for an important segment of Pistoia's people.

. . . It is at any rate certain that Pistoia's population history cannot be isolated from the changes experienced in the economy, society and culture of the medieval and Renaissance city.

PHILIP ZIEGLER (b. 1929), educated at Eton and at New College, Oxford, was for many years a member of the British Foreign Service. "I am an amateur," he writes, and not an "academic historian." His book *The Black Death* is in some ways one of the most useful works on the subject. This is not only because it has "attempted to cover every serious contribution made by students of the Black Death." The volume is enlivened by Ziegler's personal comments and the catholicity of his reading. The following selection suggests the question of whether the author's nonacademic background produced a treatment different in quality or approach from that of professional historians.*

Philip Ziegler

"Germany: The Flagellants and the Persecution of the Jews"

By 1350, the plague in France had ended or, at least, so far abated as to make possible the holding of a Council in Paris to tighten up some of the laws against heresy. But in the meantime it had moved eastwards into Germany. Central Europe was thus attacked on two sides or if, as seems probable, the Black Death also advanced by land through the Balkans, on three sides more or less simultaneously. By June, 1348, it had already breached the Tyrolese Alps and was at work in Bavaria, by the end of the year it had crept up the Moselle valley and was eating into North Germany. . . .

The details of the daily horrors are very similar to those in the cities of Italy and France and there is no need to labour them again. One point of difference is the abnormally large number of churchmen who died during the epidemic. It seems indeed that the plague fell with exceptional violence on the German clergy; because, one must suppose in the absence of other explanation, of the greater fortitude with which they performed their duties. Conrad Eubel, basing his calculations almost entirely on German sources, shows that at least thirty-five percent of the higher clergy died in this period. The figure would not be exceptionally high if it related to parish priests but becomes astonishing when it applies to their normally cautious and well protected superiors. But so far as the monks were concerned it seems that it was not only

*Reprinted from *The Black Death* by Philip Ziegler by permission of The John Day Company, Inc., publisher, and Collins, Publishers, London. Copyright © 1969 by Philip Ziegler. Pp. 84–103, 106–109. Footnotes omitted.

devotion to duty which led to a thinning of their ranks. Felix Fabri says that in Swabia many religious houses were deserted: "For those who survived were not in the monasteries but in the cities and, having become accustomed to worldly ways of living, went quickly from bad to worse . . ." The monks of Auwa are said to have moved in a body to Ulm where they dissipated the monastery's treasure in riotous living.

For a variety of reasons, therefore, the German Church found itself short of personnel in 1349 and 1350. One result was a sharp increase in plural benefices. In one area, between 1345 and 1347, thirty-nine benefices were held by thirteen men. In 1350 to 1352 this had become fifty-seven benefices in the hands of twelve men. Another was the closing of many monasteries and parish churches; a third the mass ordination of young and often ill-educated and untrained clerics. As a sum of these factors, the German Church after the Black Death was numerically weaker, worse led and worse manned than a few years before: an unlucky consequence of the losses which it had suffered by carrying out its responsibilities courageously. The many benefactions which it received during the terror ensured that its spiritual and organisational weakness was matched by greater financial prosperity, a disastrous combination which helped to make the church despised and detested where formerly it had been loved, revered or, at least, accepted. By 1350, the Church in Germany had been reduced to a condition where any energetic movement of reform was certain to find many allies and weakened opposition.

One by one the cities of Germany were attacked. As always, firm statistics are few and far between and, where they do exist, are often hard to reconcile with each other. Reincke has estimated that between half and two-thirds of the inhabitants of Hamburg died and seventy percent of those in Bremen; yet in Lübeck only a quarter of the householders are recorded as having perished. Most country areas were seriously affected, yet Bohemia was virtually untouched. Graus has suggested that this was due to Bohemia's remoteness from the traditional trade routes yet, in the far milder epidemic of 1380, the area was ravaged by the plague. An impression is left that Germany, using the term in its widest possible sense to include Prussia, Bohemia and Austria, suffered less badly than France or Italy, but such an impression could hardly be substantiated. The Black Death in Germany, however, is of peculiar interest since that country provided the background for two of its most striking and unpleasant byproducts: the pilgrimages of the Flagellants and the persecution of the Jews.

The Flagellant Movement even though it dislocated life over a great area of Europe and at one time threatened the security of governments, did not, in the long run, amount to very much. It might reasonably be argued that, in a book covering so immense a subject as the Black Death, it does not merit considered attention. In statistical terms this might be true. But the Flagellants, with their visions and their superstitions, their debauches and their discipline, their idealism and their brutality, provide a uniquely revealing insight into the mind of medieval man when confronted with overwhelming and inexplicable catastrophe. Only a minority of Europeans reacted with the violence of the Flagellants but the impulses which drove this minority on were everywhere at work. To the more sophisticated the excesses of the Flagellants may have seemed distasteful; to the more prudent, dangerous. But to no one did they seem meaningless or irrelevant—that there was method in their madness was taken for granted even by the least enthusiastic. It is this, the fact that some element of the Flagellant lurked in the mind of every medieval man, which, more than the movement's curious nature and intrinsic drama, justifies its consideration in some detail.

Flagellation as a practice seems to be almost as old as man himself. Joseph McCabe has pursued the subject with loving detail through the ages: from the Indians of Brazil who whipped themselves on their genitals at the time of the new moon through the Spartans who propitiated the fertility goddess with blood until finally he arrived at the thirteenth and fourteenth century—the "Golden Ages of Pious Flagellation." Most of these exercises were clearly if unconsciously erotic in their nature. As such, they were far removed from the pilgrimages of the Brethren of the Cross. It would be rash to assert that the Flagellants of 1348 did not satisfy, by their self-inflicted torments, some twisted craving in their natures, but "erotic," in its normal sense of awakening sexual appetites, is not a word which can properly be applied to their activities.

The practice of self-scourging as a means of mortifying the flesh seems to be first recorded in Europe in certain Italian monastic communities early in the eleventh century. As a group activity it was not known for another two hundred years. At this point, in the middle of the thirteenth century, a series of disasters convinced the Italians that God's anger had been called down on man as a punishment for his sins. The idea that he might be placated if a group of the godly drew together to protest their penitence and

prove it by their deeds seems first to have occurred to a Perugian hermit called Raniero. The project was evidently judged successful, at any rate sufficiently so for the experiment to be repeated in 1334 and again a few years later, when the pilgrimage was led by "a virtuous and beautiful maid." This last enterprise ran foul of the authorities and the maid was arrested and sentenced to be burnt at the stake. Either her virtue or her beauty, however, so far melted the hearts of her captors that she was reprieved and ultimately released.

The pilgrimage of 1260 drew its authority from a Heavenly Letter brought to earth by an angel which stated that God, incensed by man's failure to observe the Sabbath day, had scourged Christendom and would have destroyed the world altogether but for the intercession of the angels and the Virgin and the altogether becoming behaviour of the Flagellants. Divine grace would be forthcoming for all those who became members of the Brotherhood: anybody else, it was clear, was in imminent danger of hellfire. A second edition of this letter was issued in time for the Black Death by an angel who was said to have delivered it in the Church of St. Peter in Jerusalem some time in 1343. The text was identical with the first except for an extra paragraph specifically pointing out that the plague was the direct punishment of God and that the aim of the Flagellants was to induce God to relent.

The "Brotherhood of the Flagellants" or "Brethren of the Cross" as the movement was called in 1348, traditionally originated in Eastern Europe, headed, according to Nohl in a pleasant conceit for which he unfortunately fails to quote authority, by various "gigantic women from Hungary." It is to be deplored that these heroic figures quickly faded from the scene. It was in Germany that the Flagellant movement really took root. It is hard to be sure whether this was the result of circumstances or of the nature of the inhabitants. . . .

The actual mechanism of recruitment to the Brotherhood is still obscure but the appearance of the Flagellants on the march is well attested. They moved in a long crocodile, two-by-two, usually in groups of two or three hundred but occasionally even more than a thousand strong. Men and women were segregated, the women taking their place towards the rear of the procession. At the head marched the group Master and two lieutenants carrying banners of purple velvet and cloth of gold. Except for occasional hymns the marchers were silent, their heads and faces hidden in cowls, their eyes fixed on the ground. They were dressed in sombre clothes with red crosses on back, front and cap.

Word would travel ahead and, at the news that the Brethren of the Cross were on the way, the bells of the churches would be set ringing and the townsfolk pour out to welcome them. The first move was to the church where they would chant their special litany. A few parish priests used to join in and try to share the limelight with the invaders, most of them discreetly lay low until the Flagellants were on the move again. Only a handful were so high-principled or fool hardy as to deny the use of their church for the ceremony and these were usually given short shrift by the Brethren and by their own parishioners.

Sometimes the Flagellants would use the church for their own rites as well as for the litany but, provided there was a market place or other suitable site, they preferred to conduct their service in the open air. Here the real business of the day took place. A large circle was formed and the worshippers stripped to the waist, retaining only a linen cloth or skirt which stretched as far as their ankles. Their outer garments were piled up inside the circle and the sick of the village would congregate there in the hope of acquiring a little vicarious merit. On one occasion, at least, a dead child was laid within the magic circle — presumably in the hope of regeneration. The Flagellants marched around the circle; then, at a signal from the Master, threw themselves to the ground. The usual posture was that of one crucified but those with especial sins on their conscience adopted appropriate attitudes: an adulterer with his face to the ground, a perjurer on one side holding up three fingers. The Master moved among the recumbent bodies, thrashing those who had committed such crimes or who had offended in some way against the discipline of the Brotherhood.

Then came the collective flagellation. Each Brother carried a heavy scourge with three or four leather thongs, the thongs tipped with metal studs. With these they began rhythmically to beat their backs and breasts. Three of the Brethren acting as cheerleaders, led the ceremonies from the centre of the circle while the Master walked among his flock, urging them to pray to God to have mercy on all sinners. Meanwhile the worshippers kept up the tempo and their spirits by chanting the Hymn of the Flagellants. The pace grew. The Brethren threw themselves to the ground, then rose again to continue the punishment; threw themselves to the ground a second time and rose for a final orgy of self-scourging. Each man tried to outdo his neighbour in pious suffering, literally whipping himself into a frenzy in which pain had no reality. Around them the townsfolk quaked, sobbed and groaned in sympathy, encouraging the Brethren to still greater excesses.

Such scenes were repeated twice by day and once by night with a benefit performance when one of the Brethren died. If the details of the ceremonies are literally as recorded then such extra shows must have been far from exceptional. The public wanted blood and they seem to have got it. Henry of Herford records:

Each scourge was a kind of stick from which three tails with large knots hung down. Through the knots were thrust iron spikes as sharp as needles which projected about the length of a grain of wheat or sometimes a little more. With such scourges they lashed themselves on their naked bodies so that they became swollen and blue, the blood ran down to the ground and bespattered the walls of the churches in which they scourged themselves. Occasionally they drove the spikes so deep into the flesh that they could only be pulled out by a second wrench.

But though, gripped as they were by collective hysteria, it is easy to believe that they subjected their bodies to such an ordeal, it is impossible to accept that they could have repeated the dose two or three times a day for thirty-three days. The rules of the Brotherhood precluded bathing, washing or changes of clothing. With no antiseptics and in such grotesquely unhygienic conditions, the raw scars left by the spikes would quickly have become poisoned. The sufferings of the Brethren would have become intolerable and it seems highly unlikely that any Flagellant would have been physically capable of completing a pilgrimage. The modern reader is forced to the conclusion that, somewhere, there must have been a catch. Possibly the serious blood-letting was reserved for gala occasions, such as that witnessed by Henry of Herford. Possibly two or three victims were designated on

each occasion to attract the limelight by the intensity of their sufferings. The Flagellants were not fakes but some measure of restraint there must have been.

Certainly there was little in their chanting intrinsically likely to lead to total self-abandonment. The celebrated Ancient Hymn of the Flagellants, even in the Latin or vernacular German, was a pitiful little dirge; as remote from ecstatic excitement as a Women's Institute Choir's rendering of "Abide With Me":

Whoe'er to save his soul is fain,
Must pay and render back again.
His safety so shall he consult:
Help us, good Lord, to this result . . .
—Ply well the scourge for Jesus' sake
And God through Christ your sins shall take . . .
Woe! Usurer though thy wealth abound
For every ounce thou makest, a pound
Shall sink thee to the hell profound.
Ye murderers and ye robbers all,
The wrath of God on you shall fall.
Mercy ye ne'er to others show,
None shall ye find, but endless woe.
Had it not been for our contrition
All Christendom had met perdition . . .

The Flagellant Movement, at first at least, was well regulated and sternly disciplined. Any new entrants had to obtain the prior permission of their husband or wife and make full confession of all sins committed since the age of seven. They had to promise to scourge themselves thrice daily for thirty-three days and eight hours, one day for each year of Christ's earthly life, and were required to show that they possessed funds sufficient to provide 4d [deniers, pennies] for each day of the pilgrimage to meet the cost of food. Absolute obedience was promised to the Master and all the Brethren undertook not to shave, bathe, sleep in a bed, change their clothes or have conversation or other intercourse with a member of the opposite sex.

The entrance fee ensured that the poorest members of society were barred from the Brotherhood; the strict rules, at first at any rate conscientiously observed, kept out the sensation-mongers who wished only to draw attention to themselves or to give unbridled scope to their passions. In these conditions, the public were generally delighted to receive the visits of the Flagellants and, at a small charge, to meet their simple needs. Their arrival was an event in the drab lives of the average German peasant; an occasion for a celebration as well as for the working off of surplus emotion. If the plague was already rife then the visit offered some hope that God might be placated, if it had not yet come then the penance of the Flagellants was a cheap and possibly useful insurance policy. Without at first being overtly anti-clerical the movement gave the villager the satisfaction of seeing his parish priest manifestly playing second fiddle if not actually humiliated. Ecclesiastics had no pre-eminence in the movement; indeed, in theory, they were forbidden to become Masters or to take part in Secret Councils, and the leaders of the movement prided themselves upon their independence from the church establishment.

So bourgeois and respectable, indeed, did the movement at first appear that a few rich merchants and even nobles joined the pilgrimage. But soon they had reason to doubt their wisdom. As the fervour mounted the messianic pretensions of the Flagellants became more pronounced. They began to claim that the movement must last for thirty-three years and end only with the redemption of Christendom and the arrival of the Millenium. Possessed by such chiliastic convictions they saw themselves more and more, not as mortals suffering to expiate their own sins and humanity's, but as a holy army of Saints. Certain of the Brethren began to claim a measure of supernatural power. It was commonly alleged that the Flagellants could drive out devils, heal the sick and even raise the dead. Some members announced that they had eaten and drunk with Christ or talked with the Virgin. One claimed that he himself had risen from the dead. Rags dipped in the blood they shed were treated as sacred relics. All that was lacking to give the movement the full force of a messianic crusade was a putative Messiah. Such a figure had appeared in the thirteenth century but, though there may have been one or two local claimants, no major figure emerged on this occasion to lead the Brethren of the Cross into the Millenium.

As this side of the movement's character attracted more attention, so a clash with the Church became inevitable. Already the claim of the Masters to grant absolution from sins infringed one of the Church's most sacred and, incidentally, lucrative prerogatives. A number of dissident or apostate clerics began to secure high office in the movement and these turned with especial relish on their former masters. The German Flagellants took the lead in denouncing the hierarchy of the Catholic Church, ridiculing the sacrament of the eucharist and refusing to revere the host. Cases were heard of Flagellants interrupting religious services, driving priests from their churches and looting ecclesiastical property. Other heretics—the Lollards, the Beghards and the Cellites—made common cause with them in contesting the authority of the Catholic Church.

The parallel between the Pilgrimage of the Flagellants and the preceding "People's Crusades" became more apparent. According to John of Winterthur, the people were eagerly awaiting the resurrection of the Emperor Frederick[1] who was expected to massacre the clergy and break down the barriers between rich and poor. This delectable vision fused in the popular mind with the apocalyptic ambitions of the Brethren. The movement took on a revolutionary character and began to direct the hostility of its audiences as much against the rich layman as the cleric. What was left of the merchants and nobles now deserted the movement in disgust, leaving the extremists free to direct its passions as they wished.

The loss of its bourgeois members in itself would probably have mattered little to the Flagellant Crusade. But as they trekked from plague centre to plague centre, often bearing infection with them to those whom they were supposed to succour, it was inevitable that many of their older members should perish, including the responsible leaders who had set the standards for the rest. To make up numbers, pilgrims were recruited less remarkable for their piety or their dour asceticism than for their failure to fit into any regular pattern of life. Bandits too discovered that a convenient way to enter a guarded town was to tack themselves on to the tail of a Flagellant procession. Little by little the more respectable citizens of Europe began to look with diminished favor on their turbulent visitors.

Up to the middle of 1349, the Flagellants had things pretty much their own way. Central and southern Germany was their favoured hunting ground but they spread freely over Hungary, Poland, Flanders and the Low Countries. In March they were in Bohemia; April, Magdeburg and Lübeck; May, Würzburg and Augsburg; June, Strasbourg and Constance; July, Flanders. Their numbers were for-

---
[1] Probably the Holy Roman Emperor Frederick I (Barbarossa) (1152–1190). — Ed.

midable and their needs often strained the resources of their hosts. A single monastery in the Low Countries had to provide for 2,500 pilgrims in a matter of six months; in two and a half months, 5,300 Flagellants visited Tournai; when the crusade arrived at Constance it was even claimed that there were 42,000 men in the company. If anyone opposed them their reaction was ferocious. Mendicant friars in Tournai who objected to their pretensions were dismissed as scorpions and Antichrists and, near Meissen, two Dominicans who tried to interrupt a meeting were attacked with stones and one of them killed before he could escape.

From the start, however, a few doughty spirits had declined to be intimidated. The magistrates of Erfurt refused entry to the Flagellants and neither from the Brethren themselves nor from the citizens was there any attempt to defy their ruling. Archbishop Otto of Magdeburg suppressed them from the start. In Italy they made little impression; perhaps the example had not been forgotten of Uberto Pallavicino of Milan who, in 1260, hearing that a Flagellant procession was on the way, erected three hundred gibbets outside his city. The hint was taken and the pilgrims never came. In France they were beginning to gather popular support when Philip VI, showing unusual determination, prevented their penetrating beyond Troyes. . . .

They are only known to have held one ceremony in London, on the open plot in front of St. Paul's. They seem to have met with indifference or even hostility and were rapidly deported as unwanted guests.

But the turning point came with the declaration of war by the Church. In May, 1348, Pope Clement VI had himself patronised ceremonies involving public flagellation within the precincts of his palace at Avignon but he took fright when he saw that he could not control the movement which he had encouraged. Left to himself he would probably have turned against them sooner, but members of the Sacred College prevailed on him to hold his hand. In mid-1349, the Sorbonne was asked for its opinion and sent to Avignon a Flemish monk, Jean da Fayt, who had studied the phenomenon in his homeland. It seems that his advice was decisive. Shortly after his arrival, on 20 October, 1349, a papal Bull was published and dispatched to the Archbishops. This was followed by personal letters to the Kings of France and England. The Bull denounced the Flagellants for the contempt of Church discipline which they had shown by forming unauthorised associations, writing their own statutes, devising their own uniforms and performing many acts contrary to accepted observances. All prelates were ordered to suppress the pilgrimages and to call on the secular arm to help if it seemed necessary.

That the Pope meant business was shown when a party of a hundred Flagellants arrived in Avignon from Basle. Clement promptly interdicted public penance and prohibited their pilgrimages under threat of excommunication. Emboldened by his example, the rulers of Europe turned on the Brethren. Manfred of Sicily threatened to execute any Flagellant who appeared in his lands; Bishop Preczlaw of Breslau made threats reality and had a Master burned alive. The German prelates took up the attack with especial relish. The Flagellants were denounced from the pulpit as an impious sect and harsh penalties were threatened against any who failed to return humbly to the bosom of the Church. Even those who obeyed were likely to find themselves in trouble if they had played a prominent part in the movement and

hundreds were incarcerated, tortured or executed. In 1350, many Flagellants were in Rome enjoying a busman's penance by being beaten in front of the High Altar of St. Peter's.

The Brethren of the Cross "vanished as suddenly as they had come, like night phantoms or mocking ghosts." The movement did not die, indeed it was still to be encountered in the fifteenth century, but, as a threat to society or an additional headache to those grappling with the problems of the Black Death, it had effectively ceased to exist.

It is easy to poke fun at these misguided fanatics. Their superstitions were ridiculous, their practices obscene, their motivation sometimes sinister. But before condemning them one must remember the desperate fear which drove the Flagellants into their excesses. These were men who put themselves to great pain and inconvenience; in part, certainly for the sake of their own souls and their own glory, but in part also in the hope that their sacrifice might induce God to lift from his people the curse that was destroying them. There were few saints among them but, on the whole, they were not bad men. And it is impossible not to feel some sympathy for the person who, when disaster threatens, tries to do something to oppose it, however futile, instead of waiting, in abject despair, for death to strike him down.

They did achieve something. In some at least of the towns they visited they brought about a spiritual regeneration, ephemeral, no doubt, but still real while it lasted. Adulterers confessed their sins, robbers returned stolen goods. They provided some diversion at the places along their route and left behind them a fleeting hope that their pain might bring an end to the greater sufferings of the plague-striken. But when the Flagellants had passed, often leaving new centres of infection in their wake; when the miracles did not happen, the sick did not recover, the plague did not pass; then the condition of those they left behind them must have been even worse than before they came. On the whole they probably did more harm than good.

One thing at least it is hard to forgive. In his Bull condemning them, Pope Clement VI complained that "most of them . . . beneath an appearance of piety, set their hands to cruel and impious work, shedding the blood of Jews, whom Christian piety accepts and sustains." The persecution of the Jews during the Black Death deserves special attention. The part which the Flagellants played in this repugnant chapter was only occasionally of the first importance but it was none the less barbarous for that.

When ignorant men are overwhelmed by forces totally beyond their control and their understanding it is inevitable that they will search for some explanation within their grasp. When they are frightened and badly hurt then they will seek someone on whom they can be revenged. Few doubted that the Black Death was God's will but, by a curious quirk of reasoning, medieval man also concluded that His instruments were to be found on earth and that, if only they could be identified, it was legitimate to destroy them. What was needed, therefore, was a suitable target for the indignation of the people, preferably a minority group, easily identifiable, already unpopular, widely scattered and lacking any powerful protector.

The Jews were not the only candidates as victims. In large areas of Spain the Arabs were suspected of playing some part in the propagation of the plague. All over Europe pilgrims were viewed with the gravest doubts; in June, 1348, a party of Portuguese pilgrims were said to be poisoning wells in Aragon and had to be given a safe conduct to get them home. In Narbonne it was the English who were at one time accused. But it was the leper who most nearly rivalled the Jew as popular scapegoat. The malign intentions of the leper had long been suspected by his more fortunate fellows. In 1346, Edward III decreed that lepers were no longer to enter the City of London since:

. . . some of them, endeavouring to contaminate others with that abominable blemish (that so, to their own wretched solace, they may have the more fellows in suffering) as well in the way of mutual communication, and by the contagion of their polluted breath, as by carnal intercourse with women in stews and other secret places, detestably frequenting the same, do so taint persons who are sound, both male and female, to the great injury of the people dwelling in the city . . .

But it is one thing to try to infect others with one's own disease for the sake of the extra companionship, another to spread the plague out of sheer devilry. When in Languedoc, in 1321, all the lepers were burnt on suspicion of poisoning wells, it was claimed that they had been bribed to do so by the Jews who, in their turn, were in the pay of the King of Granada. There were one or two cases, notably in Spain, where lepers suffered during the Black Death on suspicion of complicity but there do not seem to be any where the Jews were not accorded the leading role and the lepers cast as the mere instruments of their wickedness.

One reason for this was that nobody had cause for envying the lepers or economic reason for wishing them out of the way. It was very different with the Jews whose popular image was that of the Prioress's Tale:

... sustened by a lord of that contree
For foule usure and lucre of vileynye,
Hateful to Christ and to his compaignye.

In Germany, and to some extent also in France and Spain, the Jews provided the money-lending class in virtually every city—not so much by their own volition as because they had been progressively barred from all civil and military functions, from owning land or working as artisans. Usury was the only field of economic activity left open to them; an open field, in theory at least, since it was forbidden to the Christian by Canon Law. In cities such as Strasbourg they flourished exceedingly and profited more than most during the economic expansion of the thirteenth century. But the recession of the fourteenth century reduced their prosperity and the increasing role played by the Christian financiers, in particular the Italian bankers, took away from them the cream of the market. In much of Europe the Jew dwindled to a small money-lender and pawnbroker. He acquired a large clientele of petty debtors so that every day more people had cause to wish him out of the way. . . . It is fair to criticise the medieval Jews for exacting exorbitant rates of interest from their victims but it is also only fair to remember the extreme precariousness of their business, dependent on the uncertain protection of the local ruler and with virtually no sanctions at their disposal to enable them to recover their money from a reluctant debtor. To ensure their own safety the luckless Jews were forced to pay ever larger bribes to the authorities and, to raise the money for the bribes, they had to charge higher interest and press their clients still more harshly. Animosity built up and, by the middle of the fourteenth century, Shylock had been born. The Jew had become a figure so hated in European society that almost anything might have served to provoke catastrophe.

But though the economic causes for the persecution of the Jews were certainly important it would be wrong to present them as the only, or even as the principal reason for what now happened. The Jew's role as money-lender predisposed many people to believe any evil which they might hear of him but the belief itself was sincere and had far deeper roots. The image of the Jew as Antichrist was common currency in the Middle Ages. It seems to have gained force at the time of the First Crusade and the Catholic Church must accept much of the responsibility for its propagation. The vague enormity of such a concept was quickly translated into terms more comprehensible to the masses. In particular the more irresponsible priests spread rumours that the Jews kidnapped and tortured Christian children and desecrated the host. They were represented as demons attendant on Satan, portrayed in drama or in pictures as devils with the beards and horns of a goat, passing their time with pigs, frogs, worms, snakes, scorpions and the horned beasts of the field. Even the lay authorities seemed intent on fostering public belief in the malevolence of the Jews; in 1267, for instance, the Council of Vienna forbade purchases of meat from Jews on the ground that it was likely to be poisoned.

To-day such fantasies seem ludicrous. It is hard to believe that sane men can have accepted them. And yet Dr. Norman Cohn has drawn a revealing parallel between anti-Semitism in the fourteenth century and under the Third Reich. On 1 May, 1934, *Der Stürmer* devoted a whole issue to alleged murders of Christian children by the Jews; illustrating its text with pictures of rabbis sucking blood from an Aryan child. Most Germans were no doubt revolted by such vicious propaganda but Buchenwald, Auschwitz and Belsen[2] live vividly enough in the memory to save this generation from any offensive sense of superiority to its ancestors. Nor do the still more recent Chinese accusations that American airmen, in 1952,[3] showered the countryside around Kan-Nan Hsien with voles infected with *Pasteurella Pestis,* the bacillus of bubonic plague, suggest that man's infinite capacity for thinking ill of man is in any way on the wane.

The Black Death concentrated this latent fear and hatred of the Jews into one burning grievance which not only demanded vengeance but offered the tempting extra dividend that, if the Jews could only be eliminated, then the plague for which they were responsible might vanish too. There was really only one charge levelled against the Jews; that, by poisoning the wells of Christian communities, they infected the inhabitants with the plague. . . .

The emphasis on this accusation is surprising. With the exception of the Faculty of Medicine at Paris, which suggested that a minor contributory cause of the epidemic might be the pollution of the wells as a result of earthquakes, none of the contemporary experts seem to have tried to link infection with the drinking of tainted water. There were other ways of spreading the plague which must have seemed at least as plausible to medieval man. Alfonso of Cordova's vision of the infection of air by the release of a "certain confection" into a "strong, slow wind" has already been mentioned and in subsequent epidemics Jews were accused of passing around clothes taken from the dead or smearing walls and windows with an ointment made from the buboes of plague victims.

A partial explanation may be that many wells in built-up areas were polluted by seepage from nearby sewage pits. The Jews, with their greater understanding of elementary hygiene, preferred to draw their drinking water from open streams, even though these might often be farther from their homes. Such a habit, barely noticed in normal times, would seem intensely suspicious in the event of plague. Why should the Jews shun the wells unless they knew them to be poisoned and how could they have such knowledge unless they had done the poisoning themselves? This theory is supported by Tschudi who, in the *Helvetian Chronicle,* records not only that the Jews knew the wells to be contaminated by "bad, noxious moistures and vapours" but also that, in many places "they warned the people against them." If they did, the warnings seem to have gone unheeded and certainly those who received them were little disposed to feel gratitude to the Jews for their consideration.

There can be little doubt that the majority of those who turned on the Jews believed in the literal truth of the accusations against them. It might be thought that this certainty would have been shaken by the fact that Jews died as fast as Christians; probably faster, indeed, in their crowded and unhealthy ghettoes. But the Christians seem simply to have closed their eyes to reality. Since the Jews caused the Black Death it was ridiculous to suppose that they could also suffer from it. Any appearance to the contrary was merely further evidence of their consummate cunning. . . .

But though such crude suspicions might

---

[2] These are three of the infamous Nazi concentration camps in which millions of Jews were tortured and murdered as part of Adolf Hitler's "final solution." (Hopefully this note is superfluous even for the reader of the 1970s.)—Ed.

[3] During the course of the Korean War.—Ed.

have been acceptable to the mob, they can hardly have been taken seriously by the intelligent and better educated. Dr. Guerchberg has analysed the attitude of the leading plague tractators. The most remarkable feature is how few references there are to the guilt or innocence of the Jews. Konrade of Megenberg brusquely dismissed the accusations: "Some say that this was brought about by the Jewish people, but this point of view is untenable." In his *Buch der Natur* he cites as evidence Jewish mortality in Vienna which was so high that a new cemetery had to be constructed. Gui de Chauliac was equally categoric. Alfonso of Cordova considered that, by all the rules of planetary action, the Black Death should only have lasted a year and that any subsequent extension must be the result of a wicked plot. But he did not specifically accuse the Jews of being responsible. The "Five Strasbourg Physicians" warned against poisoned food and water but it is doubtful whether they believed that the poisoning was done deliberately by man. No other tractator paid any attention to the possibility that some human agency was involved in the spread of the plague, still less that such villains must be identified as the Jews.

On the whole, this reticence on the part of the tractators must be taken to indicate that they did not believe the accusations. It is impossible that they did not know what had been suggested and, if they had really thought that a principal cause of the plague was the poisoning of the wells by Jews, then they could hardly have failed to say so in their examination of the subject. Their silence might imply that they thought the idea too ridiculous to mention but it is more likely that they shrank from expressing publicly an unpopular view on an issue over which people were dangerously disturbed.

For it took considerable moral courage to stand up for the Jews in 1348 and 1349 and not many people were prepared to take the risk. The first cases of persecution seem to have taken place in the South of France in the spring of 1348, and, in May, there was a massacre in Provence. Narbonne and Carcassone exterminated their communities with especial thoroughness. But it is possible that the madness might never have spread across Europe if it had not been for the trial at Chillon in September 1348 of Jews said to have poisoned certain wells at Neustadt and the disastrous confessions of guilt which torture tore from the accused. Balavignus, a Jewish physician, was the first to be racked. "After much hesitation," he confessed that the Rabbi Jacob of Toledo had sent him, by hand of a Jewish boy, a leather pouch filled with red and black powder and concealed in the mummy of an egg. This powder he was ordered, on pain of excommunication, to throw into the larger wells of Thonon. He did so, having previously warned his friends and relations not to drink the water. "He also declared that none of his community could exculpate themselves from this accusation, as the plot was communicated to all and all were guilty of the above charges." Odd scraps of "evidence" were produced, such as a rag found in a well in which it was alleged that the powder, composed largely of ground-up portions of a basilisk, had been concealed. Ten similar confessions were racked from other unfortunates and the resulting dossier sent to neighbouring cities for their information and appropriate action.

So incriminating a confession settled the doubts or perhaps quietened the consciences of many who might otherwise have felt bound to protect the Jews. On 21 September, 1348 the municipality of Zürich voted never to admit Jews to the city again. In Basle all the Jews were penned up in wooden buildings and burned alive. "In the month of November began the persecution of the Jews," wrote a German chronicler. Henry of Diessenhoven has recorded the movement of the fever across his country. In November 1348 the Jews were burnt at Solothurn, Zofingen and Stuttgart; in December at Landsberg, Burren, Memmingen, Lindau; in January, Freiburg, Ulm and Speyer. At Speyer the bodies of the murdered were piled in great wine-casks and sent floating down the Rhine. In February it was the turn of the Jews at Gotha, Eisenach and Dresden; in March, Worms, Baden and Erfurt.

In most cities the massacres took place when the Black Death was already raging but in some places the mere news that the plague was approaching was enough to inflame the populace. On 14 February, 1349, several weeks before the first cases of infection were reported, two thousand Jews were murdered in Strasbourg; the mob tore the clothes from the backs of the victims on their way to execution in the hope of finding gold concealed in the lining. In part at least because of the anti-Semitism of the Bishop, the Jews of Strasbourg seem to have suffered exceptionally harshly. A contemporary chronicle puts the grand total of the slaughtered at sixteen thousand—half this would be more probable but the Jewish colony was one of the largest of Europe and the higher figure is not totally inconceivable.

From March until July, there was a lull in the persecution. Then the massacre was renewed at Frankfurt-am-Main and, in August, spread to Mainz and Cologne. In Mainz, records one chronicler, the Jews took the initiative, attacked the Christians and slew two hundred of them. The Christian revenge was terrible—no less than twelve thousand Jews, "or thereabouts" in their turn perished. In the North of Germany, Jewish colonies were

relatively small, but their insignificance was no protection when the Black Death kindled the hatred of the Christians. In the spring of 1350, those Jews of the Hansa towns who had escaped burning were walled up alive in their houses and left to die of suffocation or starvation. In some cases they were offered the chance to save themselves by renouncing their faith but few availed themselves of the invitation. On the contrary, there were many instances of Jews setting fire to their houses and destroying themselves and their families so as to rob the Christians of their prey.

Why the persecutions died down temporarily in March, 1349, is uncertain. It could be that the heavy losses which the Black Death inflicted on the Jews began to convince all those still capable of objectivity that some other explanation must be found for the spread of the infection. If so, their enlightenment did not last long. But the blame for the renewal of violence must rest predominantly with the Flagellants. It is difficult to be sure whether this was the work of a few fanatics among the leaders or merely another illustration of the fact that mass-hysteria, however generated, is always likely to breed the ugliest forms of violence. In July, 1349, when the Flagellants arrived in procession at Frankfurt, they rushed directly to the Jewish quarter and led the local population in wholesale slaughter. At Brussels the mere news that the Flagellants were approaching was enough to set off a massacre in which, in spite of the efforts of the Duke of Brabant, some six hundred Jews were killed. The Pope condemned the Flagellants for their conduct and the Jews, with good reason, came to regard them as their most dangerous enemies.

On the whole the rulers of Europe did their best, though often ineffectively, to protect their Jewish subjects. Pope Clement VI in particular behaved with determination and responsibility. Both before and after the trials at Chillon he published Bulls condemning the massacres and calling on Christians to behave with tolerance and restraint. Those who joined in persecution of the Jews were threatened with excommunication. The town-councillors of Cologne were also active in the cause of humanity, but they did no more than incur a snub when they wrote to their colleagues at Strasbourg urging moderation in their dealings with the Jews. The Emperor Charles IV and Duke Albert of Austria both did their somewhat inadequate best and Ruprecht von der Pfalz took the Jews under his personal protection, though only on receipt of a handsome bribe. His reward was to be called "Jew-master" by his people and to provoke something close to a revolution.

Not all the magnates were so enlightened. In May, 1349, Landgrave Frederic of Thuringia wrote to the Council of the City of Nordhausen telling them how he had burnt his Jews for the honour of God and advising them to do the same. He seems to have been unique in wholeheartedly supporting the murderers but other great rulers, while virtuously deploring the excesses of their subjects, could not resist the temptation to extract advantage from what was going on. Charles IV offered the Archbishop of Trier the goods of those Jews in Alsace "who have already been killed or may still be killed" and gave the Margrave of Brandenburg his choice of the best three Jewish houses in Nuremberg, "when there is next a massacre of the Jews." A more irresponsible incitement to violence it would be hard to find.

Nor were those rulers who sought to protect the Jews often in a position to do much about it. The patrician rulers of Strasbourg, when they tried to intervene,

were overthrown by a combination of mob and rabble-rousing Bishop. The town-council of Erfurt did little better while the city fathers of Trier, when they offered the Jews the chance to return to the city, warned them quite frankly that they could not guarantee their lives or property in case of further rioting. Only Casimir of Poland, said to have been under the influence of his Jewish mistress Esther, seems to have been completely successful in preventing persecution.

An illustration of the good will of the rulers and the limitations on their effective power comes from Spain. Pedro IV of Aragon had a high opinion of his Jewish subjects. He was therefore outraged when the inhabitants of Barcelona, demoralised by the Black Death and deprived, through the high mortality and the flight from the city of the nobles and the rich, of almost any kind of civic authority, turned on the Jews and sacked the ghetto. On 22 May, 1348, he sent a new Governor to the city and gave orders that the guilty were to be punished and no further incidents allowed. A week later he circularised his authorities throughout the Kingdom ordering them to protect the Jews and prevent disturbances. By February, 1349, the new Governor of Barcelona had made no progress in his search for those responsible. King Pedro grew impatient and demanded immediate action. In a flurry of zeal a few arrests were made, including Bernal Ferrer, a public hangman. But the prosecution in its turn was extremely dilatory. Six months later no judgement had been passed and, in the end, it seems that Ferrer and the other prisoners were quietly released.

Meanwhile, in spite of the King's injunctions, anti-Jewish rioting went on in other cities of Aragon. There was a particularly ugly incident in Tarragona where more than three hundred Jews were killed. Here again Pedro demanded vengeance and sent a commission to investigate. The resulting welter of accusation and counter accusation became so embittered that virtual civil war ensued. In the end this prosecution too was tacitly abandoned. But the King did at least ensure that a new ghetto was built and intervened personally on behalf of several leading Jews who had been ruined by the loss of their houses and documents. When the next epidemic came in 1361 the Jews appealed to the King for protection and an armed guard was placed at the gates of the ghetto.

Flanders was bitten by the bug at about the same time as the Bavarian towns. "Anno domini 1349 sloeg men de Joden dood" [In the year of the Lord 1349 men slew the Jews dead] is the chronicler's brutally laconic reference to massacres that seem to have been on a scale as hideous as those in Germany. In England there were said to be isolated prosecutions of Jews on suspicion of spreading the plague but no serious persecution took place. It would be pleasant to attribute this to superior humanity and good-sense. The substantial reason, however, was rather less honourable. In 1290, King Edward I had expelled the Jews from England. Such few as remained had little money and were too unobtrusive to present a tempting target. Some small credit is due for leaving them in peace but certainly it cannot be held up as a particularly shining example of racial tolerance.

The persecution of the Jews waned with the Black Death itself; by 1351 all was over. Save for the horrific circumstances of the plague which provided the incentive and the background, there was nothing unique about the massacres. The Jews had already learned to expect hatred and suspicion and the lesson was not one which they were to have much opportunity to forget. But the massacre was exceptional in its extent and in its ferocity; in both, indeed, it probably had no equal until the twentieth century set new standards for man's inhumanity to man. Coupled with the losses caused by the Black Death itself, it virtually wiped out the Jewish communities in large areas of Europe. . . . It is a curious and somewhat humiliating reflection on human nature that the European, overwhelmed by what was probably the greatest natural calamity ever to strike his continent, reacted by seeking to rival the cruelty of nature in the hideousness of his own man-made atrocities.

Professor of the history of economics and political economy at the University of Munich, FRIEDRICH LÜTGE (b. 1901) is one of the leading scholars in the field of German economic, agrarian, and social history from the Middle Ages to the present. The following selection from his volume on *German Social and Economic History* derives from a major article on "The Fourteenth/Fifteenth Century in Social and Economic History" (1950) which directly influenced the course of subsequent German scholarship on the Black Death.*

Friedrich Lütge

Germany: The Black Death and a Structural Revolution in Socioeconomic History

The impulse which released new developmental tendencies resulted from more than a further concentration of population that had caused a transition strengthening the "urban" branch of the economy. It resulted from an outside event, namely the huge population losses brought about by the Black Death. First in 1347–1349, then again in 1357–1362, 1370–1376, and 1380–1383, Germany and the whole of western and central Europe was devastated by the plague. This does not take into account the numerous regional outbreaks of plague which began before the "Great Death" and continued to carry off large numbers until into the fifteenth century, well beyond the high point of the plague.

Whether these great epidemics, seen in their entirety, caused the death of half or "only" a third (or in individual regions a smaller or higher percentage) of the population is difficult to establish, given the present state of investigation. But it is clear that the huge human losses must have had far-reaching effects on the whole social and economic structure. This was in no way extraordinary since the plague was not an isolated event that occurred suddenly and that one could perhaps endure under the traditional social and economic system. This destructive catastrophe kept repeating itself over a period of four or five decades; two generations lived under its impact. And its impact, taken altogether, was

*From Lütge, Friedrich: *Deutsche Sozial- und Wirtschaftsgeschichte*, 2. Aufl. Enzyklopädie der Rechts- und Staatswissenschaft, Abt. Staatswissenschaft (Berlin-Göttingen-Heidelberg: Springer, 1960), pp. 177–185. Translated by William M. Bowsky. Footnotes omitted.

colossal; its power is scarcely conceivable. The atmosphere of healthy optimism which marked the spirit of the age underwent a sudden change. What had happened was incomprehensible, and only if it were seen as a punishment of God or a product of the devil could it be even doubtfully understood. If this historical event deeply affected the artistic and cultural framework of the time, it could not have by-passed the more basic structures. One should therefore remain conscious of the dislocating impact the Black Death had on the forms of objective, established institutions.

The structural revolution unleashed by this catastrophe expressed itself, with regard to the economy, in a change in the traditional relations of the factors of production to one another. This was because the Black Death, unlike a war, did not destroy property. Men died but their goods remained intact. Therefore the survivors could divide among themselves the property of the deceased. This process meant a decline in production. The labor factor experienced a sharp diminution, but land and the means of production stood relatively high in relation to consumption. With consumer goods the situation was similar. In this shifting of relations lies the crucial difference between the Black Death and the second great catastrophe that Germany experienced, the Thirty Years' War [1618–1648], which destroyed not only men but also property. One may also compare Germany to contemporary France, which was wasted by the Hundred Years' War. (The probable reason why France failed to surpass its eastern neighbor in the fifteenth century was that it had to make up not only for population losses, but also for the destruction of property resulting from the war.)

The situation was further intensified because the plague struck towns more severely than the countryside. Now more than ever the towns were dependent on increased immigration from rural areas. Because of the high death rate (especially among children) the towns could not maintain themselves through their own strength. It has been estimated that the larger German cities of the fourteenth and fifteenth centuries were able to replenish only about 50 percent of each generation from their own ranks. The fact that in these centuries there was a demonstrable decline in the urban birth rate worsened the situation. The declining birth rate was probably due to the new social and economic conditions in the towns (to be dealt with below) and especially to the abnormally great age difference between numerous marriage partners during this period (for example, a young man marrying the old widow of a master craftsman and vice versa). Also extant statistical material clearly shows that the number who emigrated to the cities soared after the Black Death.

The social and economic results of these catastrophic, overwhelming events can be conceived of as the unleashing of a "dynamic of contraction," which shows itself above all in creation by the plague of a relative surplus of land with, at first, no one to cultivate it. This "dynamic of contraction" and the structural revolution caused by it—although not having the same effect everywhere—characterized itself especially in the following ways:

(a) One of the most important and also enduring results was the abandoning of settlements. The study of settlements has long ago established that numerous villages that were settled from the twelfth to the fourteenth century were later abandoned. . . .

(b) The decisive cause of the wholesale

abandonment of land lies in the heavy population losses of this time and in the agrarian crisis that was now developing. This explanation was first elaborated by Wilhelm Abel.[1] The agrarian crisis —another result of population loss— expressed itself in more than a century of declining prices for agricultural products. The decline marked a decisive change from past centuries, when there had been a steady rise in agricultural prices only temporarily interrupted by the effects of bad harvests. Above all, wheat prices, already lower than prices for meat and cattle products, dropped. The cause lay in the relative overproduction of wheat, and this was traceable to the fact that consumers died in greater proportions than production declined. Added to this was an official policy of forced labor, which certainly caused the high level of production through compelled growing. This policy failed to achieve its purpose of providing food in times of famine and merely supported overproduction. Therefore the pressure on prices remained steady, or perhaps occasionally even increased. But the price decline was not steady; it was interrupted continually by strong up-and-down fluctuations. These fluctuations produced years in which both production and prices were high. This only made for an uneven trend, however, not a rising one. The phenomenon of suddenly declining prices is clearly evident if one converts the amounts in extant price statements into actual purchasing power. By doing this one can remove the obscurity of the price decline which is caused by changes in nominal worth (debasement of coinage, etc).

(c) Along with the drop in agrarian prices there was a rise in the price of manufactured goods. Thus a "price-scissors" developed which was unfavorable to the agrarian economy. In the towns population losses had been especially great, but property had not been destroyed. The survivors fell heir to the property. Sometimes property was inherited by legitimate heirs and sometimes (as the sources often testify) abandoned property simply went to those who occupied it. Often the lord in the countryside and the municipal government in the cities confiscated heirless property. One can therefore speak of a great shift in wealth, both individual and collective. Part of the wealth consisted of money, precious metals, etc., which could be used to purchase all types of goods. Purchasing power was accordingly concentrated in the hands of the survivors. Just as this concentration of purchasing power caused a relative increase in agrarian production, so too it caused a relative decrease in the production of manufactured goods. Production of manufactured goods declined because the newly acquired wealth allowed people to live without working or by working only a little. And after the catastrophe of the Black Death survivors enjoyed unbridled self-indulgence. The new wealth showed itself in increased demand and in a readiness to sanction higher prices. The income of workers also rose, as the now scarcer journeymen were well aware of their worth. This is the time to which Werner Sombart[2] refers in speaking of two masters running after one journeyman. Culturally, the situation led to an increased production of pre-

---

[1] Abel, professor at the University of Göttingen, is the author of the most influential study of *Wüstungen*, or abandoned settlements. (See below under Suggested Additional Readings.)— Ed.

[2] Werner Sombart (1863–1941) was a German economist, perhaps best known for his study of modern capitalism, *Der moderne Kapitalismus.* —Ed.

cious luxury goods and an increase in the erection of costly buildings, etc., the results of which are still preserved today in museums and old towns. Of course the pattern described above was not typical everywhere. The rush of rural craftsmen and other rural inhabitants to a town was often greater than the town's ability to absorb the newcomers. In such cases the usual policy favoring immigration was changed into one restricting it. Nor did all crafts share in the ascendancy of urban labor described above, especially not those concerned with simple consumer goods. The luxury crafts, however, benefitted from this development. Although there was diversity in the pattern, there can be no doubt but that a strong emphasis to the towns occurred.

(*d*) Socially and economically the flowering of the towns is considered to be the most important phenomenon coloring the German economy from this time on. While the towns flourished, the peasantry and landed nobility declined. The price decline in the agrarian sector led to a reduction in the income of the rural population, and, seen in its entirety, to an alteration of the total income structure in favor of urban groups. For the first time the craftsman gained economic ascendancy alongside the merchant, who had previously dominated the town economy. As a result a change in production took place; consumer goods were supplemented or entirely replaced by luxury goods, which sold in ever-increasing quantities to a continually expanding market. The consolidation of wealth, augmented by the dissolution of individual money hoards, led to an increase in earning power, which in turn unlocked greater opportunities for profit in commerce and manufacturing.

This soon led to a strong movement of rural population to urban centers. As always it was the most resolute, the most reasoning and, incidentally, the most unscrupulous elements that emigrated. The lower classes experienced a great ascendancy, apparent even in the art of this time. "Instead of the towering forms of the thirteenth century, sculpture and painting distinctly embodied the rise of a breed of men from the lower social strata" (Alfred Weber).[3] This rise makes understandable the . . . guild revolutions, which led to a transformation of the urban constitution through artisan participation in city government; and, incidentally, it also affected the rural population, inspiring the peasants to make attempts to gain their freedom.

(*e*) The guild revolutions (guild struggles) were primarily revolts of the guild-organized artisans. They were usually revolts of the richer, more powerful craftsmen (rather than of all urban craftsmen) against the patrician regime, which had itself replaced the preceding city-lord government. Moreover, the success of a guild revolution never led to domination by all the guilds. Usually only certain of the guilds, and in some cases only one guild, actually ran the city. And these guilds did not rule alone, but in league with the patrician "families." The situation of the lesser artisans, members of the lowest social strata remained as before. Beginning in the fourteenth and fifteenth centuries these lesser artisans constituted a genuine "social question," especially in the larger cities. In the later phases of the so-called guild revolutions even these classes occasionally tried to obtain a share in running the urban regime, but without success. . . .

(*f*) The landed nobility now declined in relation to the urban world. The de-

---

[3] A German sociologist, author of *Kulturgeschichte als Kultursoziologie* (Cultural History as Cultural Sociology) (1935, 2d ed. 1950).—Ed.

cisive reason for this was perhaps also the change in the economic structure. Only in small measure did the noble (the landlord) support himself from the direct exploitation of his land; instead he depended on ground rents for the greater part of his income. But this source of income was diminishing. Numerous peasant holdings were no longer occupied. Where they were occupied, the peasant was able to lessen his obligations in many ways because he was in high demand. There was, moreover, a decline in the purchasing power of money. This especially affected rents, which were fixed in nominal units (many of them in Carolingian times). Thus the landlords became impoverished. It appears almost symbolic that one of the most important and for a long time most well-to-do groups among the landlords, namely the German knightly order, was reduced to bankruptcy. During this period an increase in the landholdings of the nobility occurred, perhaps as a result of the absorption of abandoned lands or of free allods.[4] However the increase did nothing to remedy the plight of the noble, as the value of land was continually dropping. It was only at the end of the fifteenth century, after the agrarian crisis was brought under control, that their lands began to prove of value. At first the noble sought relief by mortgaging his property. This perhaps explains why King Wenzel[5] in 1390 granted the impoverished a general remission of debts owed to Jews; among those whose debts were remitted in this manner were the knights who had mortgaged their property to urban moneylenders. At times the noble became a highwayman in order to maintain himself. Or he entered the peasant or burger class, or he took service, usually in a military or administrative capacity, with nobles who were still prosperous. Only in regions where the nobles had extensive powers of coercion over the peasantry, as in the east, was a new economic foundation laid. The new economic foundation was a manorial regime similar to that in France, whose development was likewise distinguished by an intensification of landlord rights over the peasants. In England, however, similar developments stimulated trends which led to personal and political freedom.

It would of course be one-sided to consider these economic factors as the only causes of the decline of the landed nobility. Additional causes were the dying out of many noble families, especially those of the high nobility, and the decline of the military importance of the knights. If the military importance of the knights had remained unchanged, kings and princes would probably have found ways to protect the corresponding economic importance of this class. The declining political significance of the landed nobility reversed itself after the emergence of the territorial state. The noble was then no longer bound to the ruler by reciprocal loyalty and conditions of service carrying a personal bond. Instead he had become part of the impersonal organization that characterized the territorial state.

(g) This ascendancy of the landed nobility, which accompanied the formation of the modern state, is also a part of the picture of this time. Although the territorial state did not originate at this period (its origins can be traced back to the thirteenth century), it now developed real power. It not only absorbed the noble into its impersonal organization (which

---

[4] An allod, or alod, was a property owned fully, as contrasted with a feudal fief which a person held of his lord.

[5] The Holy Roman Emperor Wenzel (of Bohemia), 1378–1400. — Ed.

reached a high point of development in the seventeenth and eighteenth centuries), but, because of the demanding need for intense regulation of the economy, it also began to control wages and prices. The protective and organizational functions, which until then had been taken care of and profited from by various landed nobles and urban governments, could, in view of the general need, be administered effectively only by an extraordinary tribunal with authority over both the towns and the countryside. The territorial ruler worked—as indeed did all Europe— for increased production. For this reason he regulated labor and issued ordinances concerning clothing, ornaments, servants, etc. Improvement in taxation put money in his hands. The funds further strengthened his power, allowing him to pay officials and a standing army. The territorial ruler strongly relied on the assistance of members of the bourgeoisie, who were then being educated at the newly founded universities.

This situation lasted until the end of the sixteenth century when the nobles, enjoying a new social, economic, and political ascendancy, replaced the bourgeoisie as the ruler's chief assistants. The bourgeoisie and the territorial state thus furthered each other's interests; this was probably an expression of a general sociological phenomenon in which the state and the bourgeoisie both tended to impersonalize and rationalize all human interaction. The nobility and the peasantry, on the other hand, emphasized the personal bond in human relations, even attaching economic obligations to it.

The joint blossoming of the urban middle class and the state was no accident. The foundation for further development, which would take place in the sixteenth century, had now been laid. The late fourteenth century was the decisive turning point. It is valid to say that new forms of social and economic life, both individual and collective, began during this period.

A professor of history at the University of Iowa, JOHN B. HENNEMAN, JR. (b. 1935) is the author of *Royal Taxation in Fourteenth Century France.* The provocative thesis that he proposes in the following selection is certain to arouse scholarly interest and stimulate a variety of investigations.*

John B. Henneman, Jr.

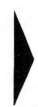

France: A Fiscal and Constitutional Crisis

The epidemic of 1348–49 known as the Black Death was a catastrophe for all of Europe, but its timing was particularly unfortunate for the kingdom of France. Long afflicted by inadequate finances and recently weakened by military defeat, the French crown had managed, late in 1347, to obtain an unusually large war subsidy from the three Estates of the kingdom. The circumstances surrounding this grant created the possibility of some future constitutional relationship between taxation and assemblies, but collection had barely begun when the plague threw all into disarray. Hopes that royal finances might be put on a sound footing speedily collapsed. With considerable effort and ingenuity the government

managed to restore some measure of fiscal stability by 1351, but it had lost the opportunity to escape from the awkward makeshift financing characteristic of the past generation. The years 1347–51 form an important background to the famous fiscal and constitutional crisis of 1355–58.[1] The precedents implicit in the 1347–48 subsidy grant would then be drawn upon, but the use of these precedents would be determined by the financial situation which developed after the plague. . . .

---

[1] These years saw the renewal of the Hundred Years' War by King Edward III of England and the invasion of France by his son, the Black Prince; abortive attempts at parliamentary control of the French government by the Estates General; and the ill-fated uprisings of the rural peasantry (the Jacquerie) and of Étienne Marcel in Paris. — Ed.

---

* From John B. Henneman, Jr., "The Black Death and Royal Taxation in France, 1347–1351," *Speculum,* XLIII (1968), 405, 412–413, 427–428. Reprinted by permission of The Mediaeval Academy of America. Footnotes omitted.

There was . . . considerable promise early in 1348 that a reformed royal government, with the collaboration of the Estates and considerable assistance from the papacy, would be able to place the crown's finances on a sound footing at last. Had this development been permitted to continue without interruption, the prestige and effectiveness of assemblies might have greatly increased. Frequent meetings at different levels in 1346 and 1347 had already produced evidence of greater experience and confidence among the Estates, with more systematic trading of troops for reforms. The trend seemed unmistakably to point towards a more effective role for a central assembly.

It was in this situation that the Black Death made its appearance, reaching Languedoc towards the beginning of Lent, 1348. By October, high mortality was reported as far north as Rouen. From such widely separated places as Rodez and Amiens we have evidence that existing cemetery space was proving inadequate. Many citizens fled the towns in panic. Our concern here is not so much with the plague itself as with its fiscal effects. It has long been accepted that the impact on taxation was considerable, but a recent demographic study by Cazelles[2] has shown that generalizations about the whole kingdom can be very risky. In the first place, the death toll may have been as much as three times greater in Lanquedoc than in the northern and central parts of the kingdom. Concentrating primarily on Languedoil [northern France], Cazelles discovered that the heaviest mortality was among children and the poorer classes of adults. This fact would imply that those most able to pay taxes were least affected

------

[2] Raymond Cazelles, a specialist in thirteenth- and fourteenth-century French political and social history. — Ed.

and that the number of taxable *hearths* did not decline sharply until a dozen or more years later when the children of 1348 would have become heads of households.

The conclusions of Cazelles thus suggest the need for caution in considering the fiscal impact of the Black Death. On the other hand, such fiscal documents as do remain for this period make it abundantly clear that the large subsidy granted in 1347–48 could not be collected. The Estates of Senlis begged to have reduced the number of men-at-arms they were committed to support. The Normans, who seem to have increased their earlier tax grant at a new assembly in May of 1348, were unable to convene in a subsequent meeting scheduled for July, and the collectors of taxes began to encounter opposition. . . .

The historian of French taxation must always labor under the handicap imposed by the destruction of the archives of the Paris Chamber of Accounts in an eighteenth-century fire. The documents which survive are widely scattered and their survival has been to some extent a matter of chance. It is perhaps risky, therefore, to attribute too much importance to fluctuations in the number of remaining documents. Nevertheless, . . . the number of surviving fiscal texts does fluctuate widely between 1347 and 1351. For the winter of 1347–48 they are fairly abundant; from mid-1348 until early 1350 there is little evidence; then the supply of documents increases, with a substantial number available for 1351. Are we not entitled, albeit cautiously, to associate this fluctuation with the Black Death? Where adequate texts are preserved, notably at Montpellier, we have ample evidence that the plague had a disastrous effect upon royal taxation. We may note in addition the wide disparity between the subsidy granted in 1347–48 and the subsidy receipts recorded at the treasury in the second half of 1349. It seems clear, therefore, that the plague, whatever its demographic effects in different parts of France, struck a crippling blow at the finances of the crown in 1348–49.

That the Black Death should have disrupted the collection of taxes is not in itself very remarkable. What is significant, for France, is the timing of the plague with respect to the constitutional development of the kingdom. The Estates of 1355 have long been regarded as a milestone, and rightly so, but there is reason to believe that their importance has been over-emphasized. But for the Black Death, the Estates of 1347 might have accomplished as much, or more, in making central assemblies respectable in France and creating the basis for constructive negotiation of taxes on a national basis. Cazelles, limiting his study to court politics, has already discovered interesting parallels between the crisis of the mid-1340's and that of the mid-1350's. It is evident that these parallels also exist in the fiscal sphere and would have been apparent but for the effects of the Black Death.

The methods employed by the crown in recouping royal finances in the aftermath of the plague are difficult to classify because of the regional variations that are always so apparent in fourteenth-century France. Yet they do suggest certain conclusions. In the case of southern France, an elaborate combination of propaganda and pressure had to be applied. This region posed a threefold problem to the crown. In the first place, Languedoc probably suffered much greater mortality than did the North. In addition, this was precisely the region where hearth taxes were customary, and yet the hearth tax was the least profitable form where the population had suffered sharp decline.

Finally, Languedoc faced the greatest military threat, even in time of nominal truce, because Gascony was the most effective base of operations for the English. Languedoc, therefore, required special treatment, and the crown rather ingeniously utilized the military vulnerability and the accession of a new king to squeeze substantial revenues from this region. Perhaps four times as much money was obtained from Languedoc in 1351 as in 1350.

If Languedoc posed special problems and tested the crown's ingenuity, Languedoil possessed a tradition of greater uniformity of taxation and greater cooperation among the Estates. This tradition was not always well marked, but the royal government would build upon it in restoring the crown's finances during the 1350's. The Estates of Languedoil, summoned by a new monarch for propaganda purposes, helped establish the pattern of taxation in northern and central France during the early 1350's. This assembly, in February 1351, expressed its loyalty to the king and acknowledged his need for financial support even in time of truce. The plague's effects seem to have been tacitly recognized in that Languedoil no longer judged taxation exclusively in terms of the military threat. No new central assembly was needed in the next few years; details could be worked out at the bailiwick level. What was important in Languedoil after the Black Death was that annual assemblies at the regional level became accustomed to trading taxes for royal concessions. No longer was the need for the tax debated; now discussion revolved around the concessions which the crown was prepared to offer. It was this experience at the local level that made possible the actions and pretensions of the French Estates General in the later 1350's.

CHARLES VERLINDEN (b. 1907) is a professor at the
University of Gand and director of the Academia
Belgica in Rome. He has written extensively on the
history of medieval markets and trade, and is the
author of the best-known study of slavery in the Middle
Ages. In the following excerpt from a major article on
the Great Plague of 1348 in Spain Verlinden concludes
that the Black Death brought about "no real changes
in the fundamental character of any political, social,
or economic institution."*

Charles Verlinden

Spain: A Temporary Setback

Let us now recapitulate the situation
which we have just described in its essential traits.

The plague spread in Spain from May
1348. Moving from east to west, it appeared first on the shores of the Mediterranean, in Catalonia, in the kingdom
of Valencia—probably also in that of
Murcia—and in the Muslim kingdom of
Granada. Then it reached Aragon and
finally Castile. It is probably this last
country which—relatively and on the
whole—suffered the least. However it is
impossible to give controllable statistics
for this.

The economic and social consequences
of the epidemic were analogous in the
different regions of Spain. They were
first felt, of course, in those areas struck

earliest by the plague. There is a chronological and geographical succession of
royal ordinances which corresponds
perfectly to the extension of the epidemic
in time and space. These ordinances were
destined to relieve the troubled situation
left in the wake of the plague. They were
promulgated in 1349 in Catalonia, in 1350
in Aragon, and in 1351 in Castile.

In Castile as well as in Catalonia, it was
first a matter of stopping the depredations
to which the masses had surrendered
themselves. Next it was necessary to control the labor problem. The primary goal
of all the legislation was to regulate prices
and salaries in a manner favorable to
employers and consumers—that is, essentially, to the privileged classes: the
urban bourgeoisie, the nobility, and the

*From Charles Verlinden, "La Grande Peste de 1348 en Espagne," *Revue Belge de Philologie et d'His-
toire*, XVII (1938), 143–146. Translated by William M. Bowsky. Footnotes omitted.

clergy. The measures were taken directly by the court in Castile and Aragon. In Catalonia, however, where royal power was weaker and the influence of the towns greater, the king merely enacted some general measures. Their application in particular cases was left to the urban authorities.

The economic pattern of agricultural and industrial work was in no way modified. No new principle was introduced. There was no hint of a decline in the corporate regime, in the sense that freedom of labor was established. Recruitment of the work force remained the same. The increase in the slave population was a general characteristic of the thirteenth, fourteenth, and first half of the fifteenth century and was not, as is believed, exclusively the result of the great pestilence. This increase was due essentially to the development of commerce with the Levant.

The abundance of legislative measures enacted to regulate the working conditions of workers and artisans proves that it was above all the masses that suffered from the plague. The rise in the price of labor cannot otherwise be explained. . . .

Nevertheless, other social classes too suffered from the plague. Though, without doubt, they were less stricken numerically, they suffered great losses with regard to their property because of the plague. This was especially true of the landed proprietors, noble and bourgeois, whose incomes diminished greatly.

The king himself did not escape the general impoverishment. He was obliged to agree to numerous tax remissions and even lost some of his properties.

Only the Church gained some advantages from the situation. Numerous donations extended its domains, and this at the very least compensated for the losses it suffered.

The great plague caused considerable disturbance in Spain but no real changes in the fundamental character of any political, social, or economic institution. If it momentarily retarded economic evolution, it did not modify the orientation of this evolution. Moreover, we believe that this is a conclusion that is valid for all of Europe.

GEORGE A. HOLMES (b. 1927), fellow, tutor, and
librarian at St. Catherine's College, Oxford University,
is a student of late medieval and early Renaissance
history. His scholarly publications include *The Estates
of the Higher Nobility in Fourteenth Century England*
(1957). Holmes's emphasis upon the decisive impact
of the plague in English history should be compared
with the views expressed in the selections from
Kosminskii and Russell.*

George A. Holmes

England: A Decisive Turning Point

A few single events in English history
have been both sudden and enormously
important. English history without the
battle of Hastings and the consequent
imposition of a new Norman aristocracy,
or without the battle of Saratoga, and the
consequent loss of the American colonies,
would be unimaginably different. The
Black Death of 1349 is a turning-point
of a different but equally decisive kind.
It initiated a long period in which the
basic material forces working on society
were different from what they had been
in the central Middle Ages, and this
change had profound effects on almost
every aspect of history in the century
after. The first plague of 1349 was un-
matched in its ferocity but it began a

long period, ending only with the Great
Plague of London in 1665, in which pestilence frequently recurred; during the
centuries of the Renaissance and Reformation men lived in terror of this common scourge. The age of plague began
quite suddenly with the Black Death and
it quickly altered the climate and tendencies of English history.

The bubonic plague, which was carried
by black rats and had already ravaged
much of the continent of Europe, probably appeared at Melcombe Regis[1] in the
summer of 1348. In that year and the next
it spread through England like a forest

---

[1] A port in southern England in the county of Dorset and diocese of Salisbury.—Ed.

* Reprinted from *The Later Middle Ages, 1272–1485* by George A. Holmes. By permission of W. W. Nor-
ton & Company, Inc., and Thomas Nelson & Sons, Ltd. Copyright © 1962 by George Holmes. Pp. 136–148.
Footnotes omitted.

fire, killing large numbers of people in every part of the country. Though we are suspicious of the hysterical entries of chroniclers, in this case they were justified; monasteries were sometimes nearly wiped out. In the diocese of Lincoln, which stretched from the Humber to the Thames, just over 40 per cent of the beneficed clergy died. In 1361 the scourge returned in the "Second Pestilence," or "Pestilence of the Children," as it was sometimes called, because it particularly attacked the young rather than those who had perhaps acquired an immunity in surviving the earlier plague; and it recurred in 1368 and 1375. After this it became increasingly frequent and also less severe, until in 1454 William Paston could write fairly calmly that he was retiring into the country to avoid an outbreak in London: plague had become one of the accepted hazards.

Apart from the catastrophic mortality of 1349 itself, the plagues caused a long decline in population. England in the reign of Edward II [1307–1327] . . . was a heavily populated country in which cultivable land was scarce. In the fifteenth century it was quite different. We do not know exactly how much of this change was due to the plague; the great floods and famines of the years 1315–17 had perhaps been the turning-point which ended the medieval expansion of population. In the over-populated England of 1315 many people must have lived on plots of land which could barely support them, or on barely adequate wages, so that they were very vulnerable to any natural calamity. Population growth may have been halted by the natural limits of subsistence. But there is little doubt that plague was the main factor in causing a steep fall in population. No one compiled population statistics in the Middle Ages, but we can tell from the changes in wages and prices that men must have been scarcer in the fifteenth century. And there are also the tangible evidences of abandoned villages. It is quite likely that a population of about 3½ millions in the early fourteenth century had been reduced to 2½ millions by the sudden and then gradual fall lasting into the mid-fifteenth century. After that the population probably began to grow again, but only slowly; soon after 1500 a Venetian visitor was struck by the fact that "the population of this island does not appear to bear any proportion to her fertility and riches," and it was probably not before the reign of Elizabeth I that as many people lived in England again as had done in the reign of Edward II.

It would be a great mistake to suppose that English society was quickly crushed by this series of disasters. On the contrary there are many reasons for thinking that in the reign of Richard II (1377–99) it blossomed in a profusion of original activity such as it had never known before. Chaucer and Langland were writing the masterpieces, the *Canterbury Tales, Troilus and Criseyde,* and *Piers Plowman,* which made English a great literary language after its centuries of obscurity. The naves of Winchester and Canterbury, the choir of York, and Westminster Hall were being built. The Wilton Diptych, perhaps the most beautiful medieval English painting, was made for Richard II. Wycliffe and the Lollards were attempting to resurrect apostolic religion. The cloth industry was growing and English merchants, masters of their own trade as never before, were thrusting into the Baltic. In almost everything from perpendicular architecture to cloth export the civilisation of this country was more distinctively English, less bound to the common hierarchy and heritage of Christendom, than it had been for centuries.

But, while the break-up of Christendom continued, the artistic and cultural blossoming of English civilisation did not. The wider diffusion of wealth and education in fifteenth-century England probably meant that a higher proportion of the population could read books and buy works of painting and sculpture than in 1300. The music of John Dunstable, who served in the household of John, Duke of Bedford, in the minority of Henry VI, the beautiful bronze effigy of Richard, Earl of Warwick, set in his memorial chapel at Warwick later in the same reign, or the chapel of King's College, Cambridge, begun by Henry VI, would be outstanding in any period. But these are almost the only aesthetic peaks and they do not equal the achievements of the age which saw the rebuilding of the octagon at Ely and the choir at Gloucester, or those of the reign of Richard II. Fifteenth-century art was more widely spread but also less impressive in individual examples. The churches of Somerset and other flourishing wool and cloth areas reached a new level of general excellence and lavishness in parochial architecture. The commonest sculptural remains are the alabaster reliefs of religious subjects and the funeral brasses which were produced in large quantities and tended to become monotonously standardised. Most English painting after the Wilton Diptych is both derivative and unexciting. Social explanations of art history are full of pitfalls, but it is worth while speculating about these changes. The old centres of patronage and inspiration, the court, the cathedrals, the monasteries, and the noble households, were all weakened in their relative economic power, and there were thus fewer incentives of the kind which produced the really aspiring enterprises of the central Middle Ages. The wider diffusion of wealth meant probably more art but also less art of superlative quality. Great things of course were being accomplished on the Continent, some of them not far from England, in the age of Donatello and the Van Eycks, contemporaries of Henry VI. But English social change reduced the old sources of patronage without replacing them by new ones comparable with the Florentine merchants of the Medici period, the contemporary Flemish merchants, or the court of the Dukes of Burgundy. If Florentine humanism and the Florentine and Flemish art of this period had so remarkably little impact on England it cannot have been because they were inaccessible: the two worlds existed side by side with much political, ecclesiastical, and commercial intercourse. It must have been because there were few people with the initiative or the power to take a serious interest in them. It is impossible to escape the feeling that England in the fifteenth century was culturally dull, flat, and unenterprising and had less to compare with the inventiveness of the Italian cities than in the lifetime of Edward I [ruled 1272–1307].

The interest of this later period consists, then, less in its few immediate cultural achievements than in the profound and gradual evolution of society and politics which was turning medieval into Tudor England. In most aspects of society we shall notice these two phases, both of which are intimately connected with the changes brought about by the plague: firstly, the atmosphere of crisis, social conflict, and lively self-consciousness which characterises the end of the fourteenth century; secondly, the stability and sleepiness of a society which had quenched the fires of upheaval but was gradually changing in its essential character.

In many parts of England today there are deserted villages, places which we know from the records to have been villages in the Middle Ages and where the outlines of the houses and streets can sometimes still be seen. They are not rare; in Lincolnshire, which was one of the counties where medieval rural expansion most overreached itself, there are over a hundred discovered sites. Probably there were two different periods in which this depopulation took place and two different reasons for it. In the decades following the Black Death many villages, especially those where the land was less suited for agriculture, must simply have died out. At Woodeaton near Oxford, for instance, soon after the Black Death, the Abbot of Eynsham could persuade the few remaining tenants to stay only by reducing their rents. Later, some time in the fifteenth century, a new kind of depopulation started. Landlords, affected by the scarcity of labour and the demand for wool and meat, began to destroy villages deliberately by putting an end to arable cultivation and turning the land over to grazing for sheep or to parks for deer. In the reigns of Henry VII and Henry VIII this was regarded as a scandal and legislated against, but most of the damage had probably been done before 1485. In 1506 it was said that

about eighty years before, Pendley [in Hertfordshire] was a great town [the word means "village" in medieval English]. . . . There were in the town above 13 ploughs beside divers handicraftsmen, as tailors, shoemakers and cardmakers with divers other. The town was afterwards cast down and laid to pasture by Sir Robert Whittingham who built (Pendley

Manor) at the west end there as the town sometime stood. . . .

As early as 1459 a chantry priest of Warwick called John Rous was agitating against the destruction of villages that he had observed in the country around. "The sons not of God but of Mammon," who caused it, found wool and meat more profitable to produce than grain. The basic cause behind it was that there were many fewer people in the English countryside than there had been in the thirteenth century, and many places which had once been busy villages either naturally became, or could profitably be turned into, fields or wastes. Much of England had relapsed into economic decay, but the same factors gave new opportunities to the grazier and the enclosing landlord.

These were the long-term material results of the fall in population. The plagues also had important effects on the structure of rural society because they altered the relationship between land and labour. The seignorial society of the central Middle Ages had thrived on an abundance of men and a shortage of land which kept people bound to their plots and subjected to their landlords. It was now undermined. The most immediate effect of the Black Death, as it appeared to the seignorial lord, was to make labour scarce and wages high. In parliament the Commons, representing people of the gentry and "franklin"[2] classes, complained bitterly of the hardships resulting from this and sought measures to counteract them. Their main weapons were the Statutes of Labourers, which from 1351 onwards prescribed maximum wages and insisted that all able-bodied landless men must work. For some years the legis-

---

[2]Freeholding. One of Chaucer's *Canterbury Tales* is, of course, "The Franklin's Tale."—Ed.

lation was enforced by special Justices of Labourers in whom the Commons took a particular interest, as they did in urging increased severity in the penalties. Some of the cases show that there was competition between lords for labour and, though wages were kept lower by these statutes than they would otherwise have been, they still rose.

At Theydon Garnon in Essex about 1390

Simon Jakeboy withdrew John Pretylwell from the service of Thomas Mason into his own service in the occupation of maltmonger giving him 26 shillings and eightpence and food and clothing every year excessively contrary to the statute, which John Pretylwell formerly was a ploughman.

The period of panic and desperate measures, marked particularly by the statutes of 1351 and 1388, was succeeded by a long period in the fifteenth century when most wages were substantially higher than they had been in the early fourteenth century and the fact was accepted.

The changed conditions were manifested more seriously in a shortage of tenants. The pressure on land had been so great that many landlords found it easy to fill up the vacant holdings after the plague of 1349. By the end of Edward III's reign [1327–1377], however, the continued shortage was beginning to have its effects. Most manors had some houses and plots which were empty "by reason of the pestilence." This made things difficult all round for the manorial landlord. His tenants could now find alternative accommodation or employment and therefore he could not keep up his rents. At the same time he now had fewer villeins to perform labour services and so became even more dependent on the expensive wage labour. On top of this the tendency at this period was for agri-

cultural prices to keep low (because fewer people were buying food), while the prices of imported things and manufactures went up. Landlords, and especially manorial landlords, were hard hit. The reaction of many of them was to make the most of their ancient rights of manorial jurisdiction. Villeins, at least, could legally be compelled to stay on the manor and even to pay rent for holdings they did not want. The steward of the Earl of March wrote to a reeve of a manor in 1391 ordering him to look after the villeins lest the lord should be "disinherited of their blood." The Abbot of St Albans on his extensive estates insisted that no land should pass between his tenants by their simply making charters granting it to each other outside his manorial courts, lest he should lose control of it. The manorial system became more resented as the tenants became more conscious of their scarcity value. In the first parliament of Richard II's reign (1377) the Commons complained at length of villeins conspiring together to withdraw their services. This evident conflict of interests was lifted directly into the political sphere by the "poll taxes" of 1377–81. These were levied on everybody by head, instead of falling more heavily on the wealthy and hardly at all on the mass of the population, as did the traditional lay subsidies. The last and most obnoxious of them provoked the first social revolution in English history.

The Peasants' Revolt began at the end of May 1381 with risings on each side of the Thames at Brentford in Essex and Gravesend in Kent. The two bands of rebels converged on London and entered the city on 13th June 1381. For two days the aldermen were cowed, the court besieged in the Tower, and the city given over to the mobs. Many houses were plundered and burned; they destroyed

John of Gaunt's[3] manor of the Savoy (he wisely slipped across the border into Scotland when the revolt started); Simon Sudbury, Archbishop of Canterbury and Chancellor, was captured in the Tower and killed. For the time being the court could survive only by negotiating, and so there took place the two extraordinary interviews between the fourteen-year-old King Richard II and the rebels. The meeting at Mile End, at which he conceded the abolition of villeinage, probably took place while the rebels were entering and sacking the Tower. The next day he went to Smithfield to meet another gathering headed by the Kentish leader Wat Tyler, who presented the most extreme of the proposals. When these demands had, with what seems now a pathetic irony, been granted, the Mayor of London, William Walworth, who was riding with the King, pulled Tyler from his horse and the rebel captain was immediately slain. Miraculously Tyler's followers accepted the King's order to disperse. Whether they believed they had really won their dream, whether the death of Tyler took the heart out of them, or whether they were tired of the rebellion, at any rate the crisis at London was virtually at an end.

In both Kent and Essex the original risings were directed at least partly against the hated poll tax, but it soon appeared that the aims of the rebels were more fundamental. The charter which they extorted from the King at Mile End abolished villeinage and laid down that the annual rent of land should be no more than fourpence an acre. This probably represented in an abbreviated form the hopes of the mass of the rebels. It does not appear to have been essentially a revolt of landless men but rather of ten-

ants wishing to be rid of the irksome burdens of villeinage and the manor. William atte Marsh of Mose in Essex, who was fined along with the other tenants of the manor for his part in the revolt and had to pay twenty shillings to get back his villein holding plus his other twenty acres, was typical of thousands of men of substance in the village communities of south-east England who took part in the great "Rumor." Another set of demands, which are said to have been presented to the King by the rebels at Smithfield, are quite different.

And then . . . Wat [Tyler] rehearsed the points which were to be requested and asked that there should henceforward be no law except the law of Winchester [probably the police regulations of Edward I's Statute of Winchester[4]] and that there should be no outlawry in any process of law henceforward, that no lord should have lordship but that there should be proportion between all people, saving only the lordship of the king; that the goods of holy church ought not to be in the hands of men of religion, or parsons or vicars, or others of holy church, but these should have their sustenance easily and the rest of the goods be divided between the parishioners; and there should be no bishop in England but one, no prelate but one and all the lands . . . of the possessioners should be taken from them and divided between the commons, saving their reasonable sustenance to them; and that there should be no villein in England or any serfdom or villeinage, but all to be free and of one condition.

This proposed a total subversion of the hierarchy of society, not the ordinary villein's demand for release from the disabilities of his condition. It is clearly connected with the famous couplet of John Ball, the preacher who was condemned after the revolt.

---

[3] An extremely powerful magnate, John of Gaunt, Duke of Lancaster, was a son of Edward III and an uncle of Richard II. — Ed.

[4] A statute of 1285 that helped to create a police system. — Ed.

When Adam delved and Eve span
Who was then a gentleman?

Each of these social aspirations had a long ancestry. The desire to abolish villeinage had been foreshadowed in many village disputes between lords and tenants trying to establish "ancient demesne" (that the estate in question had been held directly by the king at the time of Domesday Book[5]), which was commonly held to free a manor of some of the burdens of unfreedom. The egalitarianism of Ball is foreshadowed in earlier sermons. The combination of the two made a particularly explosive mixture, the fight for material advantage fired with religious enthusiasm. The social circumstances—intensified conflict of interest between lords and tenants—were ideal; so was the political situation of a boy king hedged about by suspected counsellors, an unsuccessful war, a tax thought to be monstrously unjust.

The original movements in Kent, Essex, and London inspired others. In Hertfordshire, where the great abbey of St Albans covered much of the county with its manors and judicial liberties, a conscientious abbot, Thomas de la Mare, had caused much resentment by his careful guarding of the abbey's rights. On the day of the meeting at Smithfield a body of his tenants marched to London, secured from the King a charter of their rights, and marched back the same day to present it to the abbot. For some days the abbey was in a state of siege. The tenants believed there was a lost charter of King Henry I which granted them all they wished. Since it could not be found —and indeed did not exist—they insisted instead on rights of way and of hunting the woods, fishing the river, the right

to grind their own corn at home instead of in the abbot's mill, the right to buy and sell land amongst themselves and, of course, the abolition of villeinage. For a few days they lived in the delusion that their new liberty was permanent. . . .

By the end of June the revolts were everywhere suppressed. Concessions granted to buy off the rebels were withdrawn and society had returned to its previous stable hierarchy. The rebels achieved practically nothing. Their deeds are interesting mainly for their drama and for their revelation of the acute tensions in society. The social crisis of the early part of Richard II's reign died down and was succeeded by the gradual changes of the fifteenth century.

The problems of manorial and village society remained after the revolt and continued to be intensified by the growing shortage of men. The villein who flees from his native village to throw off the shackles of serfdom and live in freedom and prosperity in a distant town is a familiar legendary figure in English history. In the reigns of Richard II and Henry IV he was no legend but a real and common type. It was possible for some villeins to live legally outside their manors by paying "chevage" annually to the lords. Others simply disappeared, for the shortage of men was so great that they could easily find employment in a town or a free holding in another village, and rural society was so fragmented that it was generally impossible to recapture them. In 1387 at Wilburton in Cambridgeshire the court roll of the manor tells us that no tenant can be found for the lands which a certain villein "abandoned in flight." This was a common occurrence and its effects on the organisation of the manor were serious. Holdings had to be let to new tenants for smaller rents and often without the old labour services. The total

---

[5] The famous survey of England ordered by William the Conqueror in 1086.—Ed.

value of the rents of most manors declined somewhat and the combined effect of high wages, disappearing labour services, and low prices of grain was to make the working of the demesne lands relatively unprofitable except to provide food for home consumption.

Most of the great seignorial landlords reacted to these circumstances by giving up the direct cultivation of the demesne and leasing it to farmers. It was the accepted remedy for the difficulties of the times. The auditors of John of Gaunt said of two of his manors in 1388:

The husbandry of Higham Ferrers and Raunds is of no value beyond the costs there which are so great each year that the said husbandry is a great loss to my lord, wherefore the demesne lands ought to and can be leased at farm as in other places.

In the reigns of Richard II, Henry IV, and Henry V (1377–1422) this was happening all over England. John of Gaunt's manors, which made up the great Duchy of Lancaster, had practically no land in demesne by 1399 when his son conquered the throne. The estates of the Bishop of Winchester were all farmed out in the early fifteenth century. By 1422 the old regime of the manorial lords was practically dead.

It is more difficult to say what replaced it. The elaborate organisation of the great estates of the thirteenth and fourteenth centuries produced a mass of written records, especially accounts and court rolls, which tell us much about the manors and about the countryside in general. In the fifteenth century when lords were no longer cultivating the demesnes themselves, their manorial accounts commonly became brief lists of rents paid by tenants, and this is an obstacle to our understanding of the countryside. There are, however, a few things which we can say about

it with a fair degree of certainty. Firstly the class of substantial peasants or farmers flourished greatly and to a large extent the control of most villages was given over to them. At Forncett in Norfolk there were eighteen villein families in the manor in 1400. Six of them were still there in the early sixteenth century, of whom three continued to hold moderately sized lands while three others became big farmers: the villein family of Bolitout included one individual farming seventy-eight acres, a member of the Dosy family held two houses and a hundred and ten acres in 1500, and a Bole in 1477 farmed the whole of a neighbouring manor. Similar changes happened in most parts of England. The big farmers inherited the position of the manorial lords. This happened partly because of the leasing-out of the demesne, which put much more land at the disposal of tenants, partly also because of the shortage of tenants which enabled the more energetic of those who remained to take over vacant holdings. The typical farmer of the fifteenth century held a patchwork of pieces of land; the symmetrical villein tenements, all of the same size and owing the same services, which had been common still in the fourteenth century, became rare. The extremes of wealth and poverty in the peasantry were stretched. At Frisby in Lincolnshire in 1381 there were sixteen families, all tenants, of whom the richest were reckoned to be two or three times as wealthy as the poorest. In 1524 there were only ten families of whom three had no land and two were wealthier than all the rest together.

The second thing which certainly happened was the gradual disappearance of villeinage. The reason for this was generally not deliberate manumission of individuals (Henry VII manumitted all villeins on Crown estates in 1485 partly because villeinage was by then becoming an anomaly) or commutation of services. It was firstly because many villein families died out and could not be replaced; secondly, because many fled and their villeinage was forgotten; thirdly, because the splitting-up of demesnes made labour services out of date. In this way both personal villeinage and villein tenure gradually died. The mass of descendants of the villeins were coming to hold their lands not by the old customary tenures but by copyhold, that is to say by an agreement with the lord of the manor, made in the manor court, to which the title deed was "copy of court roll." In the reign of Edward IV [1461–1483] the common law-courts were beginning to hear cases about copyhold and the importance of the manorial court was evaporating with the rest of the manor.

JOSIAH C. RUSSELL (b. 1900), professor of history at Texas A & I University, is the outstanding medieval demographer. His classic study *British Medieval Population* (1948) opened new areas of investigation which are now being explored by scholars in America and Europe. This selection from an article on the preplague population of England is an imaginative combination of social and economic history with demographic techniques.*

Josiah C. Russell

England: Preplague Population and Prosperity

Sometime in the period 1300–48, English population reached its high point in the Middle Ages. All agree that it rose rapidly in the thirteenth century and dropped catastrophically in 1348–77. Its course in the first half of the century, however, is the subject of two sharply divergent opinions. One is that population increased gradually to about 3,700,000 at the outbreak of the plague, a point at which "the agricultural people were being crowded."[1] The other opinion[2] is less exact: population reached its height about 1315, when the great famine and pesti-lence of 1315–17 reduced the population markedly and started a decline, restrained perhaps by a mild recovery in the two decades before 1348. According to this second theory population was much denser than the 3,700,000: even in the late thirteenth century, England had a "starving and over-populated country-side," with "the poor sokemen[3] of Lincoln-shire—[struggling] to support five people on five acres of land," and "a society in which every appreciable failure of harvests could result in large increases in deaths in a society balanced on the margin of subsistence." . . .

---

[1] This is Russell's own theory.—Ed.

[2] Michael M. Postan is one of the leading exponents of this second opinion according to Russell.—Ed.

[3] Sokemen were freemen possessed of a right in the soil but subject to the court jurisdiction of a feudal lord.—Ed.

---

*From Josiah C. Russell, "The Preplague Population of England," *The Journal of British Studies*, V (1966), 1, 10–21. Most footnotes omitted.

The evidence of the years, 1310–19, shows a halt in population increase in England and the loss of perhaps a few per cent. The continental evidence of 1300–47 varies from showing a brisk advance in Sweden to showing a heavy loss in the mountains of Provence. In general the rapid increase of the thirteenth century came to an end, a plateau was reached, and the trends were local or regional rather than continental. Little evidence comes from the lands across the Channel from England, and other evidence illustrates conditions of areas unlike the English. Quite a variety of data, however, offers indications about the course of English population then.

The evidence showing that the peasants' expectation of life was much like that of the fiefholders suggests that their experience was similar in other ways. Thus since the number of fiefholders' children was sufficient to provide an increase beyond the number of their parents in the first half of the fourteenth century, it seems probable that the serfs' children also exceeded the number of their parents. Two other methods show the same increase: a comparison of numbers of people in thirty places in the poll tax of 1377 and in extents[4] before the plague, and a comparison of size of about 152 places in Domesday and in the extents before the plague. Using either the poll tax or Domesday as a base, the ratios of the extent figures to them increase

[4] The extents were descriptions of manors that listed tenants according to their positions in society: freemen, villeins or serfs, cottars or cottagers.—Ed.

throughout the preplague period. If 1. is taken as the value for the 1377 poll tax populations, the two show the increase by double decades as [shown in the table below.] Except for the high level of 1330–47, the comparative evidence from Domesday shows a lower figure than for the poll tax–extent comparison, presumably from lack of data about new villages. These show roughly a 3 per cent increase for each decade.

Direct clues about population change should be provided by comparison of extents of manors before the famine-pestilence of 1315–17 and after. One complication is that fourteenth-century extents are not as informative about population as earlier ones, frequently giving sums returned by freemen or cottars instead of numbers of these classes. As usual there are problems of identifying manors with common names. Such as have been identified mostly come from the southwest of England and, as might be expected, show little change. In Cornwall, Helston in Trigg increased slightly, as apparently did Westaford in Dorset and Curry Mallet in Somerset. In the county of Gloucester where much more evidence occurs, Fairford and Brimmesfield increased, Tewkesbury held even, while Alweston, Kingsham, and Southorp declined. Bagworth, Lechlade, and Paynswick present problems. In Hampshire, Itchel increased slightly, and in Wiltshire, Aystone and Cyriel declined. The increase is slight. To the northeast, merchets on the manors of Spalding Priory show 219 in 1276–1300, 325 in 1301–25, and 351 in 1326–50, thus

Ratio		*1290–1309*	*1310–29*	*1330–47*
Of extents to poll tax:	medians	1.25	1.38	1.45
	means	1.38	1.43	1.50
Of extents to Domesday:	medians	1.07	1.10	1.64
(D.B. = .5)	means	1.19	1.26	1.53

increasing in numbers in spite of its being a period of emancipation.

From Taunton in the southwest of England comes information about the payment of tithingpenny from male serfs over the age of twelve from 1209 to 1330 when it became standardized. It is alleged that "the central authorities, fearing the continuation of the downward trend," froze the payments. Furthermore, the author says "that there are indications that these famines, 1315, 1316, 1317, mark the turning point in the population trend." The trend of payments is susceptible to another interpretation. From an average number of 1,125 in the years 1268–78, the payments arose slowly and erratically to an average of 1,154 in the years 1306–09. In the next year, 1310, the number jumped suddenly to 1,344 and remained at about 1,337 until 1317. Then it declined to 1,202 in 1319 and from this point averaged about 1,224 until 1330. The last years of this period showed payments for 1,206, 1,221, and 1,228, which should not have disturbed authorities as a "decline." Actually the increase of the average of the years 1319–30 over that of 1306–09 was about the normal 3 per cent a decade. If one views the unexplained increase of the years 1310–16 as ephemeral, the famine hardly marks a turning point, even at Taunton.

An approach to the study of population change in this period by way of data about economic alterations suggests that "they can be found in series sufficiently consecutive and sufficiently comparable to enable us to do what direct demographic methods cannot do, i.e. to form a judgement of the continuity and duration of the trend."[5] Population data are so scarce at best that any new light upon demo-

graphic conditions is welcome, especially when offered with some assurance. "The data of wages and those of rents and vacancies agree in placing the beginning of the decline somewhere in the first twenty years of the fourteenth century." Another source is land values, but for the preplague period there is only the statement that "at the Abbey of Glastonbury, the entry fines, having risen from less than a pound per virgate in the early thirteenth century to above £12 in 1345, began to fall again after that date." Since presumably land values rise with increase of population, by this index it arose until about 1345, somewhat after the first two decades of the century. But perhaps other evidence would support the earlier period.

"Of the various categories of economic evidence capable of reflecting population trends the fullest and clearest, as well as the most neglected, is that of wages." By lumping agricultural wages in periods of twenty years, of which two are 1300–19 and 1340–59, both of which include rather sharp changes in wages, the study shows agricultural wages rising steadily in terms of agricultural prices. Presumably this indicates decline of population from about 1300. If, however, one examines the decennial averages of wages for workers in wheat (probably the commonest of wage earners) compared with the value of silver money, a different interpretation is possible. Wages varied much as did prices of wheat from 1261 (and especially from 1281) until about 1321, because workers were often paid in wheat. Then the price of wheat jumped, even in comparison to the other grains. From about 1321 wages seem to have followed the value of silver in their steadiness. If unvarying wages (in terms of wheat) accompanied an increase of population from 1261 to 1321, why should not the unvarying wages (in

[5] The quotations in this and the following paragraph are from an article of Michael M. Postan (1950). – Ed.

terms of silver) also have been accompanied by a population increase from 1321 to 1348?

The evidence of economic conditions, as yet presented, does not seem sufficient to cause one to suspect the theory of a sharp break only after the great plague and to substitute a change of population direction about 1310–19. The other evidence, with the exception of certain cities and villages, suggests a very gradual increase to 1348. It is clear that a plateau of population was reached in England before the Black Death, offering demographers and others an opportunity to study population conditions in a state of equilibrium.

Probably the best source of information about population in medieval England is the poll tax of 1377, which was to be paid by all persons over the age of thirteen, except members of the mendicant orders and manifest beggars. An estimate is made as follows:

Laity in the poll tax	1,355,555
Add 50% for children	677,778
Estimate for Cheshire	15,503
Estimate for Durham	13,091
Clergy in the poll tax	30,641
Estimate for mendicant friars	2,590
Add 5% for indigent and untaxed	104,758
	2,199,916

In general the Exchequer expected that all tax assessments be paid and was very efficient in this respect.

The collection of the poll tax of 1377 apparently proceeded like any other tax, efficiently and without objection. It was followed by a second and heavy tax two years later and a third, three times as large as the 1377 tax, in 1381. By English custom, repetition a second and a third time within a short period created a strong precedent for the future, a prece-

dent in this case for a large and regular direct tax. No wonder the people revolted. The failure to pay the 1381 tax, however, has been used to suggest that the 1377 tax may also have been avoided widely. It raises the question of the nature and purpose of the reductions in the collection of the 1381 tax. Even though the officials failed to collect a third of that tax, it still brought into the Exchequer twice as much as did the 1377 collection.

The arrangements for the payment of the 1381 tax caused ill feeling. In each district persons were to pay one shilling on the average: the rich to pay more and the poor less. This requirement placed much discretion in the tax officials. Its implication might well be that, if poor people could pay less, poor towns and even poor counties also might pay less than the official amount. If a definite pattern of evasion appears, then apparently the officials had even the 1381 tax collection under control. One complaint, indeed, was that the officials forgave some and omitted others. The officials naturally had with them the returns of the 1377 tax, returns both of the tax collected and the number of payers. In terms of numbers of taxpayers Lancashire paid on 35.1 per cent of the 1377 number, Cornwall 35.2 per cent, Cumberland 40.1 per cent, and Devon 45.3 per cent. The English probably would have said that these counties paid seven, eight, and nine shillings on the pound in comparison with the earlier tax. Shropshire and Somerset paid 55.3 per cent and 55.6 per cent. Seven counties cluster about the three-quarter point and a large number about the two-third mark. The sheriffs of the four neighboring counties of Worcestershire, Herefordshire, Oxfordshire, and Warwickshire collected 80–82.8 per cent of the 1377 number. One can almost see them agreeing among themselves to take from four fifths of the earlier number, or a little more, to avoid being obvious.

Another approach to the problem of those exempted or missed in the poll tax of 1377 is through the percentage of married persons, since the unmarried more probably escaped paying. The percentage of married would seem to be about 66–68 per cent, which would be about 44–45 per cent of the total population. If, however, the 2 per cent of the clergy and 5 per cent allotted to the exempt or missed are included, the percentage of the married drops to about 41–42 per cent which is a reasonable percentage. The plague's age specific mortality tended to be higher for the older people, many of whom were unmarried. This fact not only reduced the percentage of the unmarried but also opened the way in many cases for younger people to take land and marry. The plague, however, also prevented the number of children from increasing rapidly, keeping the percentage of those under fourteen at about the usual place. All of these approaches seem to show that 5 per cent was a reasonable figure to cover the exempted and those who escaped paying the poll tax of 1377.

The most obvious way to test the reliability of the 1377 poll tax collection would be to check its returns against contemporary documents, such as court rolls or other taxes. These documents are much less satisfactory as a check than might be expected. Persons in the court rolls, for instance, might come from other villages, be under age, or appear with different names. And probably anyone of enough means to pay another tax would also pay the rather small poll tax.

The size of the preplague population of England is reached more easily by comparison with the poll tax figures than

with the Domesday figures. The poll tax was nearer in time and avoids the problem of new villages. From the poll tax returns the preplague population may be calculated in two ways: by adding to the 1377 total the estimated losses from 1348 to 1377, and by comparing the population of the towns in the tax with the preplague extents to produce a curve of development. Both lines, starting with 2,200,000 in 1377, lead to about 3,700,000 in 1347. The decline of about 40 per cent from 1347 to 1377 is typical of European experience of the time. The estimate for the 1347 population of England secured by comparing extent evidence with Domesday, since it does not make allowance for new towns, is less than the other estimate. In the use of the extents the size of the index figure assigned to the tenement is of very great importance. By medieval standards there is considerable evidence for estimating it.

Earlier it has been shown that the extent with its inclusion of large numbers of cottars and women presupposes a relatively small index[6] for the tenement. Now evidence from about one hundred villages and cities of 1377 shows a 2.3 figure for the taxpayers to the household and thus about a 3.5 total to the tenement. Furthermore, in nineteen places after 1350 the relationship of units in extents to poll tax figures can be shown, a relationship which again indicates a 3.5 household, assuming a household to the tenant. While it has been suggested that 3.8 persons to a tenement might be proper before the plague, evidence of murder of whole households before the plague in a variety of places indicates again about 3.5 persons. The relationship of persons in thirteenth-century life tables

---

[6] By index Russell means the number of persons inhabiting one holding. — Ed.

would also indicate a 3.5 household if the holder regularly got his holding at about eighteen to twenty-three years of age, which seems to have been the case on the Winchester manors. There are enough instances of a figure this low on the continent to show that it was possible there, although in general the index for the tenement was higher there.

Another approach to the problem of the household or tenement is through its relationship to total population. The latter can be estimated from its relationship to the larger cities of the kingdom, a relationship which has been of more interest to modern regionalists than to medievalists. Nevertheless, it can be of great significance because of the essential unity of medieval agricultural life with its relatively few special centers based on mining or manufacturing which might disrupt the normal pattern of functional centers of regular occurrence. Thus in a region the size of England, the largest city might be expected to have approximately 1.5 per cent of the total population. London had in 1377 a population of about thirty-five thousand persons, which should have made it a center of about 2,330,000, a figure close to the 2,200,000 of England with some of Wales added. The secondary cities of England do not reach the size expected in the usual pattern and thus do not suggest an England larger than what is estimated for it. The centralization of English culture was such that one may not hazard, as for the Carolingian Empire, that its primitive character permitted a center of less than average size. As estimated by this city-region relationship, the total population is consistent with estimates based upon tenements of 3.5 persons rather than of a larger size.

Higher estimates of household size are based upon evidence from four places,

three of them on the Prior of Spalding's manors. For all of them wide assumptions, subject to severe doubt, concern the actual size of the household. For Spalding's manors there are lists of children of serfs: the serfs are only a part of the inhabitants of the villages. No wives are named: every tenant is given one. The households can be separated with difficulty, since men still appear as sons in one list and fathers in another, even though some names thought to be in this category have been eliminated. It is doubtful if the lists of Spalding manor are different from the other two lists: all seem to be complete lists of sons and daughters. The elimination of an erroneous idea of what was meant by "with father" and "with mother" just adds to the number of households and reduces their size.[7] Of the three sets of lists only those of Moulton seem to be larger than normal.

For the manor of Taunton high estimates of 4.3 persons in 1248 and 5.9 persons in 1311 are presented[8] confidently as the size of the household. They are based on the assumptions that: (1) all of the hundred penny payments were made by persons living on the 660 agricultural tenements of the manor, (2) the sex ratio of that period was the same as that of nineteenth-century England and thus quite low, and (3) the percentage of children was also that of the nineteenth century, quite high. None of these assumptions is probable. Children of serfs often lived away from the manor and paid chevage or other fees to keep open their rights on the manor. Medieval sex ratio was usually high, often 120 men to 100 women in agricultural areas. The nineteenth century with its rapidly growing population naturally had more children

---

[7] Russell . . . believes . . . that "with mother" means with a widowed mother in a separate household.
[8] By J. Z. Titow in 1961. — Ed.

than the thirteenth century with its more slowly increasing people. Thus it is impossible to use the Taunton data, as they are used, to indicate household numbers. Another article suggesting a large household, not only for England but for all Europe, exhibits a series of untenable hypotheses, some already mentioned: that there was a uniform household for all Europe, that one village (Halughton) was typical and the other hundred villages the exceptions, that one should accept modern China as an illustration of medieval Europe with respect to social class differences in mortality, that there were a very low number of unmarried persons and a very high percentage of children in 1377, and finally that conditions of tax collecting were very similar in 1377 and 1381.

The size of English population is also associated with the question of overpopulation. Few would believe that an England of 3,700,000 would see many persons, especially on the farms, starving except perhaps in the famine years of 1315–17. What has to be shown then is that there really were periods of starvation, as alleged, each time grain prices went up. The evidence merely shows a good correlation between high prices of grain and large numbers of deaths. The obvious reason for this is that poor weather conditions, usually extreme dampness or dryness, produced both poor harvests and bad conditions of health. Death rates follow the weather throughout the year: they should normally follow conditions of particular years.

The theory of overpopulation rests in part upon a failure to consider the age and sex distribution of the population. One is told that 29 per cent of the villein tenants and 47 per cent of the free tenants have less than five acres of land. The reader naturally sees "the poor sokeman struggling to support five persons on five acres of land" and feels that one acre was not enough to support one person. However, if it is realized that one sixth (actually 17.3 per cent of a large sample) are women who would have few dependents, the picture changes somewhat. One eighth of the men retired before death on the Winchester manors, probably a fair sample of English farmers then. Between the women and the elderly men about 30 per cent of the households are accounted for. Apparently obligatory labor covered less than one half of the work on the demesne, land not included in the peasant holdings mentioned above. This need for extra labor would offer work and wages, not merely to the 20 per cent of tenants holding five acres or less (after the aged and women were set aside), but to a considerable number of persons who had more than five acres of land.

On the question of subsistence there is apparent agreement that a tenant and his family needed five to ten acres, preferably near ten. Since those who have so calculated had a family of five in mind, the subsistence base was one or two acres to a person, preferably near two. If one takes the figures prepared for a group of 13,504 landholders, free and serf, in the Hundred Rolls of 1279–80,[9] multiplying each class by a proper number of acres, one can get an estimate of the number of acres available to each person. [See table, p. 107]. This is, it seems, an average of nearly fourteen acres to the tenant, well above the margin of subsistence by any standard. It assumes nearly three acres to a person, if the family averaged five. If, however, the household averaged only 3.5 persons, each member would be

---

[9] The Hundred Rolls contained the answers to questions posed by royal commissioners to juries in all English counties in order to ascertain royal possessions and rights. — Ed.

Number of landholders	Percent	Size of holding	Average acres in holding	Total acres
510	3.8	Over a virgate	40	20,400
3,143	23.3	A virgate	30	94,290
3,448	25.5	Half virgate	15	51,720
1,474	10.9	Fourth virgate	7.5	11,055
4,929	36.5	Petty holdings	2	9,858
13,504	100.0			187,323

supported by four acres of land. In addition, a high proportion of the poor tenants would add wages from work on the demesne, probably the equivalent of another acre to the person. And five acres to the person is 2.5 times a generous minimum of subsistence. These holdings are in parts of England which did not increase much in population between 1279–80 and the Black Death. From such a high average holding, England, according to a contemporary chronicle in 1316, "once helped other lands from [her] abundance," a statement validated by data on export and import trade.

This is a natural conclusion. English documents include tenants of social classes, even women and the elderly, and thus assume a relatively low number to the tenant and household. Winchester and Spalding evidence shows that peasants had about the same expectation of life as the fiefholders, whose life tables thus seem reasonable for all of English men. Although the decade 1310–19 probably saw the loss of a few per cent, the first half of the century saw English population rise gradually, probably reaching about 3,700,000. The poll tax of 1377 was collected carefully from all but the few per cent exempted or missed. The evidence for a 3.5 household is extensive and impressive. Far from suffering from overpopulation, England was a prosperous country in all but the worst years. While the economy may have reached a plateau just before 1348, the decline came only with the plague.

In an intensive study of the plague of 1348 in an individual town, ÉLISABETH CARPENTIER contends that "the governmental, economic, and social framework of society in Orvieto successfully resisted the agony of the Black Death." The impact of the pestilence, she holds, is rather to be seen in a "demographic catastrophe," and, most especially, in "the profound trouble of individuals and souls."*

Élisabeth Carpentier

Orvieto: Institutional Stability and Moral Change

We have set ourselves the task of discovering what had changed in Orvieto after the plague, as compared with pre-plague Orvieto. We have not found any revolutionary change or permanent destruction in the different sectors that we have studied so far. In the political, administrative, and financial sectors we have observed the accentuation of tendencies that were already clear before the plague. The plague aggravated a preexisting situation; it did not cause a profound change. In the economic sector this aggravation was quite strong; it determined the great reform of 1350,[1] which

was both an enterprise of conscience and an attempt at recovery. But when we leave the realm of legislative decisions and the domain of statistics to move closer to human realities, the changes are much more tangible. We have seen some concrete examples: the impossibility of placing in order the accounts of notaries killed by the plague, the problem of relations between guardians and wards, problems that affected orphans, the many women and adolescents who were heads of families, and the great scarcity of doctors as well as of harvesters and grape gatherers. All these questions—each one

---

[1] Carpentier argues that the government of Orvieto instituted a great financial and economic reform in 1350 which included the substitution of a hearth tax for the traditional tax based on property evaluation. Although showing that the reforms already were compromised in 1351 and proved relatively ineffective, Carpentier adds elsewhere in this work that "one of the most remarkable consequences of the plague" is that "for once, Orvieto adopted an economic policy."—Ed.

---

*From Élisabeth Carpentier, *Une ville devant la peste. Orvieto et la Peste Noire de 1348* (1962), pp. 192–195, 222–225. By permission of S. E. V. P. E. N., Paris. Translated by William M. Bowsky. Footnotes omitted.

posing specific problems for specific individuals—were new. From these symptoms we can see that the lives of the Orvietans were deeply affected by the plague, even if their official institutions were not. The Orvietans who knew the plague and survived it received a shock, as investigations in the religious, moral, and psychological domains will demonstrate in detail.

It has been said and repeated, with evidence to support it, that the plague of 1348 provoked a revival of religious sentiment, or at least the outward manifestations of one. What was there of this at Orvieto? For 1348 we have found nothing special on this subject, except adoption of the religious interpretation of the plague as a divine punishment caused by man's sins. The *Riformagioni*[2] of 1349–1350 offer nothing new on the subject. The annual giving of alms by the commune to religious establishments occurred at the beginning of each year. Celebration of great feasts took place regularly, sometimes accompanied by the traditional liberation of prisoners.

There were nevertheless signs of increased religious fervor. On August 11, 1349, in a deliberation held for "the well-being, repose, utility, convenience and profit" of the people of Orvieto, the first solution proposed was of a spiritual not a material nature. In future the vigil of the Assumption was to be observed, as well as the feast of Saint Severus, the feasts of saints whose relics were preserved in the city or its suburbs, and the feasts of saints who had given their names to churches in Orvieto or in the suburbs. We have here a spectacular example of the accentuation of external manifestations of worship, for these acts amounted to the creation of at least fifty new holidays (a list of churches, dated August 17, 1350, bears sixty names, but several of the churches were dedicated to the Virgin) devoted, by definition, to religious activities. This appears to modern eyes as a strange way to remedy an economic crisis or a labor shortage, but it is very revealing of a state of mind profoundly imbued with religion.

The pilgrimage was another exterior religious manifestation. The year 1350 was a Jubilee Year and the flow of Christians toward the Holy City was large. Orvieto was not a stranger to this movement. From the first, situated as it was on the route to Rome, Orvieto offered its facilities to pilgrims, throwing open all the city gates, which had habitually been jealously kept closed and guarded. The "Historical Discourse"[3] informs us well on this subject: "The nights when the gates were closed were rare because of the numbers of pilgrims who passed through by day and by night." Moreover, the Orvietans themselves desired to go to Rome and gain Jubilee indulgences. The commune encouraged them to do this. "So that in this happy time of Jubilee, the people of the city and of the contado may more easily be able to go to Rome in order to obtain . . . indulgence . . .," it was decided on October 26 to suspend investigation and judgment on all civil cases until the following year. An analogous measure was taken on November 20 "for the convenience of the people of the city and countryside who have gone or will go to Rome for the indulgence of the Jubilee."

Construction of the cathedral continued. Although few payments were made in 1350, they were numerous in 1349; mainly attested to by the transportation of marble from the region of Pisa. The commune concerned itself particularly with the good progress and the ad-

---

[2] Records of City Council deliberations.—Ed.

[3] A chronicle of Orvieto.—Ed.

ministration of the work on the cathedral, as well as with the procurement of the necessary materials. . . . We do not know if construction of the cathedral suffered from the same labor shortage that affected other sectors of activity in Orvieto, but the nomination of a new supervisor, Vitale di Lorenzo, on June 19, 1350, testifies to the continuance of the enterprise.

Taken in their entirety, our sources reveal the existence of a normal religious life, at least insofar as official religious life was concerned. The traditional feasts were celebrated, alms were given, and work on the cathedral continued. The creation of new feasts and the Jubilee year pilgrimages to Rome even testify to a special fervor. We must ask ourselves here if these official, external manifestations of collective and individual piety were accompanied by a renewal of internal and spiritual life, expressing itself, for example, in more exacting moral demands. Austerity and penitence would supposedly have appeased the divine wrath embodied by the plague. But nothing like this took place. Orvieto in the years 1349–1350 offers an undeniable spectacle of moral laxity, which proves once again that if government, the economy, and society had succeeded in resisting the catastrophe, the individual citizens had yielded to it. Such yielding was not restricted to the laity. Ecclesiastics, decimated and discouraged by the plague, were unable to aid the population in efforts at redress, and these churchmen were the only ones who would have been able to assure the continuity and efficacy of the previous moral standard. . . .

Before, during, and after. . . . The behavior of Orvieto before the plague of 1348 now appears clearer to us. First, several difficult years prepared a terrain favorable to the epidemic. Then, at the moment that it struck—as is easy to see

from the veil of silence covering official texts—the life of the city was completely disrupted. Nevertheless, things were quickly reorganized; judging from the situation at the end of a few months, on the basis of administrative documents, one can even doubt the severity of the disaster. Finally, it is necessary to look ahead some years in order to evaluate validly the deeper consequences of the epidemic. These results, which are verified in every area, allow us to place this crisis in its proper place in the history of the fourteenth century and to answer some of the questions we posed at the beginning of this study.

On the political level, Orvieto had already for half a century been experiencing growing difficulties in both city and contado. Increasingly, it suffered pressing and repeated intervention by its neighbors, at the request of some of its own citizens. From 1337 on the civil struggles and wars became more violent than ever, only diminishing temporarily in 1348 under the influence of the plague and the stewardship of Perugia. The shock passed and strife broke out again more sharply in a psychological climate that was even worse than before. This strife ended in 1354 with the submission of the city to Cardinal Albornoz, marking the end of its independence. In fact, despite the disorganization that had paralyzed the political life of Orvieto for some weeks in 1348, the influence of the plague on events themselves appears quite minimal in the long run. It is far more important for the psychological atmosphere in which those events unfolded.

The economic sector is much more sensitive than the political sector. Already before the plague a grave economic crisis was affecting Orvieto. A series of poor harvests, caused by bad weather, provoked high prices, then scarcity, and finally famine. This was accompanied by a general rise and confusion in prices and an increase in wages, which we were able to evaluate in the case of the Priors.[4] At the same time financial difficulties disturbed the commune. The plague epoch also was marked by a momentary disorganization of commerce and by a new rise in prices. Next a general labor shortage became the major problem. But other problems accompanied it, the most notable being the rise in prices and wages as well as the weakening of the commune's money. The commune of Orvieto enacted two measures to counteract these trends. In 1348, it authorized a general price increase to a level 25 percent higher than preplague price levels. Two years later it embarked on an extensive price readjustment, permitting variable increases in different sectors. But this arbitrary reform was not sufficient to moderate a process already operating for several years and considerably aggravated both materially and spiritually by the plague. The abandonment of lands, the desertion of the countryside, the shortage of artisans and of members of the liberal professions (we have observed the situation with regard to physicians, judges, notaries, butchers, and especially peasants) checked all attempts at redress. And these phenomena, which appeared right after the plague, showed no tendency to disappear later. Sapped at its base, one can say, the economic life of Orvieto continued each year to manifest signs of persisting decline. The long-term consequences of the plague were as tragic as the immediate consequences.

On the social level the sources leave us with a greater margin of uncertainty.

At Orvieto, the first half of the fourteenth century was characterized by distinct social tension. A study of society in the town brings to light different groups which sometimes fought and sometimes allied with one another, in multiple and diverse combinations. The nobility, upper bourgeoisie, artisans, common people, and peasantry each had their own interest and history. Our sources do not allow us to speculate whether the plague struck one social class severely while sparing another. The sources that we have deal mainly with the upper bourgeoisie, which was severely hit by the plague. The percentages of dead among the Seven and the Twelve[5] are impressive. All this leads us to believe that the plague struck the majority of urban dwellers and peasants just as severely. Furthermore, in the short run the epidemic did not alter the relationship among social forces, but in the long run the nobility, deprived of its peasant work force, was the great loser. Moreover this new situation only accentuated a tendency which already was inclining nobles to the trade of mercenary soldier or to banditry. So once again the plague only accentuated and favored an evolution begun earlier.

We must recognize that on the whole, except during the months of the epidemic itself, the governmental, economic, and social framework of society in Orvieto successfully resisted the agony of the Black Death. Seen from the outside, political life, social relations, and commercial activities followed the same norms in 1350 as they had in 1346 and 1347. If one reads the sources rapidly it even seems that nothing had changed at all, that the same immutable structures continued to rule the same society. These appearances

---

[4] Carpentier here refers especially to the traditional high communal magistracy of Orvieto, the Seven, or the Seven Consuls of the Guilds.—Ed.

[5] This magistracy of the Twelve appeared in Orvieto during the plague period. Chosen by the Seven, the Twelve served together with them.—Ed.

are misleading, however. A profound study of the years 1349–1350, like the history of Orvieto in the second half of the fourteenth century, shows that even if the institutions remained the same, they now related to a population which was diminished both quantitatively and qualitatively. This was the veritable drama of the plague, and it became fully manifest only long years later.

It is absolutely necessary to repeat that the population diminished quantitatively. Because of the lack of adequate statistics, Orvieto makes only a modest contribution to the problem of plague mortality. Nevertheless the number of deceased found among the Seven, the Twelve, and notaries is high and testifies to a death rate of more than a third, or even than a half, among the groups studied. In addition, a comparison of the number of taxpayers in 1292 with the number in 1402 shows that the population of Orvieto declined by about half during the fourteenth century. One can truly speak of a demographic catastrophe, and even if institutions did not change, their context thus appears singularly modified.

Moreover, the diminution in the number of inhabitants was accompanied by a grave change in their physical and moral health. The plague of 1348, characterized by a preponderance of the pneumonic form, left aftereffects, which the survivors, cared for by an insufficient number of doctors, had to endure. In addition, for generations the people suffered new attacks of the plague, and remained menaced by it. These two essential phenomena —the brutal, constant diminution in the number of the living and the permanent menace that threatened them—profoundly affected the population and had important psychological consequences. We will not cite again the numerous sources that show the indolence, dishonesty, and

immorality existing in postplague Orvieto. There is not space to discuss the problems of individuals and families— the problem of orphans being most characteristic—which we glimpse in the sources. The plague of 1348 bequeathed a troubled situation to Orvieto. The plague of 1363 only aggravated it. On the psychological level this second outbreak was of capital importance: it let the Orvietans know that the epidemic of 1348 had not been a unique and exceptional accident, but that the menace of plague was always present. And it was in 1363 that real sentiments which had been carefully hidden in 1348 appeared openly: fear shamelessly exposed, cowardice, and at the same time the desire to profit from and even exploit the present. Certainly the Church gave the epidemic of 1348 an interpretation which the Orvietans, fervent Catholics, did not fail to adopt. But if the severe moral crisis which then developed led some to a life of penitence— the best example of this is the rise of religious brotherhoods—it did not induce all to a life of austerity, but quite the reverse. Even the members of the clergy itself suffered deeply from the consequences of the plague. Thus we meet again, on the religious and psychological plane, the opposition between the apparent immutability of general structures and the profound trouble of individuals and souls. At Orvieto at least, this opposition appears to be the great change effected by the plague of 1348.

A war, or a revolution, causes a disturbance of human institutions which leaves source material that is accessible to the historian. Battles, annexations of territory, constitutional changes, and social or economic reforms are described by contemporaries and are recorded in documents on the basis of which posterity can establish its judgments. A catastrophe such as the one of 1348 has far deeper and graver consequences than any war or revolution. Even at Orvieto, it caused more victims, in a few months, than had all the civil and military struggles which had taken place in the town and its contado for many years previously. But the epidemic attacked individuals and not their institutions. By that very fact it has not left the historian tangible proof of its gravity and importance. With regard to Orvieto, we have been able to establish the absence of immediate sources on the plague and, further, we have been able to appreciate the exceptional wealth of later documents which apparently have no precise connection with the epidemic. The contrast between the extensiveness of the phenomenon and the poverty of sources directly concerning it is not peculiar to Orvieto. It is part of the history of the plague, and can contribute to clarification of the contradictory opinions which have been expressed on this subject.

WILLIAM M. BOWSKY (b. 1930), professor of history
at the University of California, Davis, is a specialist
in late medieval and early Renaissance history. His
published works include *The Finance of the Commune
of Siena, 1287–1355* (1970). In the following selection
he suggests that while the Black Death did not disturb
communal finance to the extent that might be expected,
it did produce great economic and social dislocation
and fluidity. These factors, together with the results
of repopulation, helped to upset traditional political
norms and create the conditions that led to the violent
overthrow of the oligarchy that had governed the
commune of Siena for nearly seven decades.*

William M. Bowsky

Siena: Stability and Dislocation

By January 1349 the storm had passed
and the restoration of order was under
way. The major task fell to communal
authorities. Although important officials
had died, the disruption of the summer
had been only temporary. Communal
records show a continuity of legislative
and administrative personnel. Many
Noveschi[1] lived on to play key roles in
government, as did members of the great
noble families even though they remained
excluded from the IX.

Equally important, administrative
techniques were not seriously disrupted.
Comparison, for example, of the volume
recording the deliberations of the IX in
November–December 1347 with that for
September–October 1351 reveals continuity in the functioning of the IX, in
the nature of the issues they treated,
methods of action, and even in the format
and composition of the volumes of deliberations. In fact, the very few indications
in the 1351 volume that there had been a
major disaster are indirect. Biccherna
and City Council records demonstrate
continuity in recording and accounting
procedures. Sixty years of *Noveschi* rule
and close attention to the details of government had laid firm foundations.

---

[1] The Nine, the highest governing body in Siena
from 1287 to 1355, was an oligarchy of bourgeois and
noble origin that excluded certain great noble or
magnate families from its ranks by law. The term
Noveschi applies to those who served on the Nine
and their relatives.

---

*Revised and adapted for this volume by the author, from William M. Bowsky, "The Impact of the Black
Death upon Sienese Government and Society," *Speculum*, XXXIX (1964), 19–34. Reprinted by permission of
The Mediaeval Academy of America.

This is not to deny a shortage of personnel after the epidemic. As early as 15 August 1348 it was necessary to order that the names of the dead be removed from the lists of persons eligible to hold office on the IX. The chamberlains of Siena's two most important financial magistracies, the Biccherna and the Gabella, had hitherto been selected from among the regular clergy, most frequently from the Cistercian monastery of San Galgano. But on 22 August 1348 these offices were opened to laymen, as because of the plague it "is difficult, nay, impossible, to have any monks from any order or monastery for the said offices . . . since so few remain that they are not even sufficient in number to celebrate divine offices in their own monasteries." So severe was the crisis that contado communities received permission to select their own vicars to serve until 1 January 1349, filling out the terms of those who had died during the plague. The greatest shortage, that of judges and notaries and of foreigners to serve in such high posts as those of Podesta and Captain of the People, remained acute throughout the regime of the IX. Nonetheless, governmental machinery was rapidly re-assembled and was manned by the same type personnel as before the epidemic.

Many problems remained to be solved, including the resumption of communal income. The Black Death did not end the need to pay foreign officials and mercenaries. Siena required troops to protect her contado and to fight her wars. She had to maintain her commitments to Florence and her Guelf allies; particularly to resist the incursions of the Milanese Visconti into Tuscany. And in 1354 the pressures exerted by the fierce *condottiere*,[2] Fra Moriale, dwarfed all others.

To add to Siena's difficulties, officials and troops demanded higher wages than before the plague, both because they were in short supply and to offset any increased cost of foodstuffs. Almost all measures providing monetary bonuses for communal officials or mercenaries refer to the "immensely" increased cost of "victuals" as well as to the shortage of personnel. Legislation aimed at restricting the practice of augmenting salaries with frequent bonuses proved ineffective.

Surprisingly, Sienese finances were quickly restored and even improved. 1340–1352 the Biccherna's semestral expenditures averaged about £ 210,000. This was less than the 1341–1344 budgets (£ 260,000– £280,000), and not much above the £215,000– £ 195,000 of 1345–1348. More significant, each successive group of Biccherna magistrates needed to advance less to cover its predecessor's debts. The Biccherna's total indebtedness was less than it had been in 1330, while the total budget for that year was only half of that averaged 1349–1352.

By 1353 Siena approached that rarity, a balanced budget. This it accomplished without resorting to a devaluation of coinage and despite remissions of fees granted to gabelle[3] farmers and renters damaged by the plague. In 1354 the newfound stability was abruptly jarred when the ravages of Fra Moriale occasioned the largest budget to date in Sienese history. The Biccherna spent over £ 300,000 during the first half of that year alone.

Low forced loans and a very light tax were levied in the summer and fall of 1348. 5 December the price of salt that Sienese were compelled to purchase from

---

[2] A *condottiere* was the commander of a large mercenary band or army.

[3] Most gabelles were indirect taxes, and in Siena they were "farmed"; that is, the government (through the magistracy of the Gabella) sold these taxes to the highest bidders—bidders who would pay the government a set sum for the right to collect gabelle and keep its income themselves.

the commune was increased 25%, the first such price increase in eight years. 22 January 1349 the City Council enacted legislation that permitted the compounding of fines at 10% to 25% and the cancellation of all existing death sentences against any individual upon payment of 600 gold florins. During the first half of 1349 alone over £ 23,600 was collected from 635 persons who took advantage of the discounts and composition.

Two means were basic in the achievement of financial improvement. Indirect taxes were increased, and in many cases doubled. More important, the commune exacted forced loans in larger amounts and more frequently than ever before. Most struck the wealthier inhabitants of the city and the Masse,[4] and to a far lesser extent those of the contado. The Jubilee Year of 1350 brought new prosperity to innkeepers and others doing business along the routes to Rome. These were taxed with a forced loan of 4,000 florins. In 1353 a thousand florin forced loan was imposed on foreign money lenders doing business in Siena. During the second half of 1351 alone the commune realized over £ 75,000 in forced loans, more than £ 60,000 of which came from inhabitants of the city. Other forced loans followed, accompanied by a *dazio* (a form of direct tax) of slightly over 6% in the city. This money could be exacted because the government guaranteed repayment of forced loans by obligating specific portions of communal income, especially the gabelle on wine sold at retail in the city and contado.

Voluntary loans ostensibly repaid at a profit of 8%–10% a year apparently accounted for a share of the communal income. In actuality, though, Siena recog-

nized that many lenders received more than the legal interest rate, for the commune excused this practice if the lender paid an "excess profits tax" of 20% on the interest that he collected beyond the legal limit. Interestingly, despite any new riches that were amassed as a result of the plague, the voluntary lenders to the commune continued to be drawn principally from the same *Noveschi* and great nobles as before.

Siena did not try to strengthen itself at the expense of the contado. The annual contado assessment[5] remained at the low £ 36,000 set in 1347. This was only 50% more than the original assessment of 1291 even though expenditures had risen more than 200%.

Nor could the contado support heavy impositions. Almost all work ceased during the summer of 1348. Fields were neglected and animals left untended, as men were scarcely able to care for their own ill. Mills closed down and most were still inoperative as late as February 1349.

The death toll was high, but varied greatly from one community to the next. In 1353 the Maremma commune of Sassoforte numbered fifty men. Before the plague it had sheltered one hundred sixty men and their families. Neighboring Montemassi was reduced to less than fifty men, from a pre-plague population of two hundred and twenty.

Migration as well as plague deaths accounted for these losses. Throughout the period that we are considering, and long after, many contado lands lay sterile, unworked because of the shortage of farm labor. From 1354 on the incursions of mercenary companies increased the crime and disorder that followed the plague.

As early as September 1348 communi-

---

[4] The Masse was a name given to a group of subject communities immediately adjacent to Siena that were differentiated juridically from the contado.

[5] This refers to a sum levied on and apportioned among the communities of its contado by the commune of Siena.

ties throughout the contado barraged Siena with requests for financial assistance, particularly in the form of remission of rentals and fees owed the commune. The honesty of these petitions is attested by the fact that they were granted despite the loss of income to Siena. Siena was solicitous of the contado's troubles. It immediately remitted the one-third of the annual contado taxation due in September 1348.

Remissions and even the cancellation of contracts were also conceded to private individuals and groups of men renting communal properties in the contado. 14 August 1349 several Sienese who had rented the entire court, district, land, and castle of Marsiliana for eight years beginning 1 January 1348 for £ 5,950 (at the rate of £ 850 a year) successfully petitioned for the cancellation of their contract. They alleged that because of the plague they could not hold and use this territory, nor even guard it from Siena's enemies should the need arise. Two of the original renters had died, and, worse yet, it was impossible to find men to serve as either guards or as agricultural laborers. In June 1349 renters at Civitella Ardenghesca received a four-year reduction of one-third in the rentals due from houses and squares in the castle and from olive groves, and a 50% remission of farm rents. But even this aid was insufficient. Six months later all these Civitella contracts were cancelled at the renters' request upon the receipt of small payments.

In 1351 Siena went so far as to aid contado communities at the risk of slowing the rate of repopulation of the city itself. Wealthy men of the contado who wished to acquire Sienese citizenship were now required to notify the communities on whose tax registers they were enrolled of their intention. This was done so that the communities affected could, if they so desired, protest officially to the City Council. Nor could one obtain Sienese citizenship without first obtaining an official release from his community. This measure passed with almost no opposition, by a vote of 120 to 3.

The Sienese government recognized that *ad hoc* relief to individual communities or renters was not enough. By October 1349 the City Council granted the leading Sienese magistracies authority to combine contado communities for the purpose of the taxes and services they owed Siena. This measure was needed because some communities had been completely wiped out and others decimated. The action was taken "since because of the plague that has occurred many contado communities are reduced to nothing . . . [it is ordered] from humanity and piety . . . so that they may be kept in the service of the commune of Siena with their customary devotion and faith."

In 1350 it was manifest that a complete new reassessment of the contado communities was needed in order that the annual taxation might be imposed in an equitable fashion:

Since from the fatality that has occurred all the contado communities generally have decreased in population, but their decrease is unequal. Some have decreased moderately, others immensely, still others have been completely wiped out. Hence there results the great inequality of taxation that exists today. And since whatever is unequal is intolerable the said taxation must be returned to fitting and tolerable equality, and must be made and done anew.

In accordance with this measure the entire contado tax burden was reapportioned in relation to the damage suffered by each community.

The shortage of agricultural labor and the increased demands made by renters, sharecroppers, and farm laborers who survived the epidemic caused Siena to try to attract foreign farm labor into the state. In 1349 such immigrants were promised immunity from taxes and services until 1354 if they would farm specified amounts of land. At the same time those men aged fifteen to seventy who had customarily rented, sharecropped, and worked were heavily taxed unless they farmed the same specified quantities in the customary fashion. This law was necessary:

Since the workers of the land, and those who customarily worked the lands and orchards, because of their great extortions and the salaries that they receive for their daily labors, totally destroyed the farms of the citizens and inhabitants of the state [districtuales] of Siena and deserted the farms and lands of the aforesaid citizens and districtuales.

While this measure may have driven some peasants into foreign lands others were probably attracted to Siena itself, augmenting the city's population and labor supply. At least two other measures of 1348 and 1350 were aimed at restricting the mobility of farm laborers and compelling them to adhere to customary contracts, but they were not renewed and were apparently unsuccessful.

Those coming to Siena found a scene of considerable confusion. The epidemic was followed by an increase in the number of crimes of violence and in all forms of abandoned living. As late as 15 September 1350 the City Council lamented the ease with which culprits could evade justice merely by leaving the city.

The Black Death brought about great social and economic dislocation. Severe legislation of 1349 aimed at gaining for Siena the properties, rights, and incomes of those who had died intestate during the epidemic and were not survived by close relatives. By law those legacies pertained

to the commune, but many had been forcefully usurped. The new law provided that all who had occupied such estates denounce the fact to communal authorities within two weeks, upon pain of paying double the value of their usurpations. After the two-week grace period anyone could denounce such illegal occupation to the Podesta and receive 10% of the fine, while his name would be kept secret.

Other inheritances too were illegally seized, leaving widows and orphans to petition the City Council for redress. So numerous were contested legacies that special courts, judges and commissions were appointed to hear and define such cases. Extant testimony concerning contested dowries proves conclusively that many properties throughout the city, Masse and contado were acquired in the wake of the plague without regard to right or legal ownership.

Not all inheritances were worth accepting. Some, burdened by debt, were rapidly repudiated. The forty-one repudiations of paternal legacies approved by the City Council in 1349 are almost double the number for any preceding year.

A major cause for repudiation is found in another area of City Council activity: grants of moratoria, discounts, and remissions of fees to gabelle farmers and renters of communal properties. (The first half of 1349 saw over thirty-five such grants —more than for any previous comparable period.) So numerous were the pleas for relief that in September 1348 two separate measures were enacted establishing the administrative machinery for granting such aid to renters and gabelle purchasers damaged by a loss of income caused by the plague.

If post-plague Siena was marked by economic and social fluidity not all were losers. Sumptuary laws were quickly revived because many persons pretended to higher station than that of their birth or occupation. In legislation of 1349 knights, judges, and physicians, and their wives and children under twelve years of age were the sole groups permitted the most lavish expensive modes of dress.

Much legislation was enacted to protect the rights and properties of the multitude orphaned by the Black Death, but two closely contested measures of 9 April 1350 merit special attention. These forbade the orphans of non-nobles, particularly female, from marrying nobles without the prior consent of their bourgeois kinsmen. This was probably an attempt to protect bourgeois legacies from magnates wishing to recoup damaged fortunes or to add to existing riches. The closeness of the votes indicates clearly that not everyone accepted the new economic and social fluidity as a blessing.

Many *Noveschi* and great nobles were plague victims or bankrupted. But all wealth itself did not disappear. Some men enriched themselves with little heed to legal niceties. Others legitimately inherited sizeable fortunes. And *Noveschi* and magnates continued to lead Siena, and to lend to it, as before. Biccherna records do not bear out Agnolo di Tura's contention of 1349 that "all money had fallen into the hands of new people *(gente nuova)*."

By the fall of that year, however, enough *nouveaux riches* had come into existence, or gained sufficient strength, to cause the conservative City Council to enact a revolutionary measure: it ended forever the strict monopoly held by Sienese bankers —the core of *Noveschi* strength—over the right to act as sureties for gabelle purchasers. Henceforth non-bankers too could participate in this lucrative business, provided that the leading Sienese magistracies approved of their suitability by a two-thirds vote.

The attack on bankers' privileges was pushed further. By 1355 they were forbidden to hold two key financial offices to which laymen had gained access in 1348 because of a shortage of monks. Like the law protecting bourgeois orphans, this measure originated in the Council of the Military Companies, where lesser gildsmen held greater power than they commanded in the higher echelons of government.

Among those who gained most in social and economic status after the Black Death were the notaries. The few remaining notaries of both the city and contado profited from their scarcity. For the first time they assiduously avoided communal offices and vicarships, devoting themselves to profitable private practice and to service in the entourages of those called to high office as Podesta, Captain of the People, or War Captain. Notaries ignored both old and new ordinances regulating their fees. They even went so far as to draw up documents that were contrary to the wishes of the contracting parties, and to mock those who employed their services. In October 1352 the commune was forced to abandon its traditional policy of prohibiting clerics from practicing as notaries, even in those cases where the Gild of Judges and Notaries wished to continue the prohibition. This measure was enacted for the explicitly stated reason that notaries were in too short supply. As late as June 1354 the City Council empowered the IX to draft notaries for service in contado offices.

Plague survivors with special skills or in very short supply not unnaturally tried to improve their lot by demanding higher wages and prices, beyond what was justified by the increased cost of alimentary products. Stonemasons and others in the building industry were particularly scarce. Like other communes such as Orvieto and Pisa, Siena enacted wage and price regulations. Detailed Sienese ordinances have not survived, but there is proof that on 1 October 1348 the Consuls of the Merchant Gild received authority from the City Council to set both rates and the fines for contravention. The alleged reason for this measure was that artisans and workers were demanding far more than the customary amounts for their wares and labors. Of greater interest, though, is the fact that Siena apparently enacted only three such regulatory measures—two immediately after the plague and a third in March 1350. Even these were not renewed.

If unlike many other European communes and states Siena did not rely heavily upon such controls to restore normalcy, another avenue was open: encouragement of immigration to the city. Possibly on 13 October 1348 the government extended Sienese citzenship to those foreigners who came to Siena with their families and remained for five years. But this is only hinted at in an apostil and in a brief phrase recording a City Council vote.

If the Sienese government wished to attract new inhabitants to the city this allegedly was not to be at the expense of the contado communities, as we have seen from the legislation of 1351 restricting the ease with which wealthy contadini could obtain citizenship. Yet the law itself was probably occasioned by contado complaints against just such an exodus.

What of actual figures? In point of fact the number of new citizenships granted from September 1348 to April 1355 soared 22.5% over the total number granted during the eighteen years from 1330 to 1348. Enjoyable though it is to deal in percentages, the numbers at stake are a modest eighty and ninety-eight citizenships.

After the plague, as before, over half of the new citizens came from the contado and most of the remainder from neighboring Tuscan states. Prominent among those whose occupations are known were notaries, merchants, and wool manufacturers.

Any major influx of population after the Black Death came not at this citizen level but from the lower economic and social strata, the strata hardest to trace in extant documents. Substantial indirect evidence points to just such an influx, and to a considerable repopulation of the city perhaps as early as 1351. Such a population increase might explain in part the rapid restoration of Sienese finances. Similarly, the farm labor legislation of May 1349 was conducive to driving agricultural labor off the farms, and, to some extent, towards Siena itself. The legislation of May 1351 assisting contado communities to control the exodus of wealthy contadini wishing to acquire Sienese citizenship would not have been necessary had there been no such phenomenon. Noteworthy too is Siena's rapid abandonment of wage and price regulations for city artisans and workers, particularly as other communes such as Pisa and Orvieto long continued their use. While as late as February 1350 applicants for Sienese citizenship requested exemption from the statutory requirement that they build new houses in the city or suburbs for the specific reason that many houses were empty because of the plague and "the city needs inhabitants, not houses," such statements appear in no later applications. Not to be overlooked are the hitherto unnoticed expenditures for several new gates and walls for the city totaling almost £ 3,000 during the first half of 1352. By March 1353 the Council of the People, reduced one-third after the plague, was restored to its original size. This, coupled with the fact that the *Noveschi*-dominated City Council remained reduced, may indicate the social and economic level of many of the new arrivals.

Returned refugees may account for some of the repopulation. Some immigrants came from the Sienese contado, still others from outside the state. But while post-plague Siena housed both *nouveaux riches* and newcomers of modest means these groups were new and unstable elements in the city's political life. And they shared in certain attitudes, if not a clearly formulated program. Neither group accepted with equanimity traditional *Noveschi* methods of government—*nouveaux riches* from a desire for political and social perquisites commensurate with their improved economic status; newcomers to the city because they had not grown up under the rule of the IX.

Their attitudes coincided most closely in hostility to the special privileges and advantages that the *Noveschi* assumed for themselves. Some of these had been criticized occasionally in the past. Now the attacks became so severe that the government took cognizance of the protests and yielded in part. In June 1349 the chief magistrates of the Biccherna were attacked for favoring their friends in the priority of repayments to communal creditors and for allowing speculation in the public debt. It was less than three months later that the bankers lost their monopoly over the right to act as sureties for gabelle purchasers.

Pressures increased noticeably during the next three years. In the fall of 1350 the IX were ordered to stop receiving and giving gifts. 22 April 1351 the City Council enacted legislation aimed at eliminating suspicions that the tax assessors were favoring members of the IX, the chief magistrates of the Biccherna and the Gabella, the Consuls of the Merchant Gild, and their families. The following 8 July the IX were denied the right to elect themselves or any other incumbent leading Sienese magistrates to any public office.

So great was the pressure that eleven days later the City Council considered a proposal to enlarge the base from which members of the IX were selected—the first such proposal to reach the council floor in fifteen years. But the IX were not prepared to admit defeat. Although this measure was sponsored by a leading *Noveschi* it failed by a vote of 82 to 45. This reversal is all the more significant when we recall that the council approved over 99% of the measures that it considered.

The IX continued to see their position threatened. Accused of mismanagement of the public mint, in June 1351 one group of the IX was even deprived of its special immunities against ordinary criminal prosecution. Two months before the fall of the government Sienese bankers were explicitly excluded from two important financial offices.

The Black Death did not directly precipitate the overthrow of the IX. But it was instrumental in creating demographic, social, and economic conditions that greatly increased opposition to the ruling oligarchy. At the next major crisis, the arrival in Siena of the Emperor Charles IV in March 1355, newcomers and new rich were important elements in the revolution that felled a government that had weathered the storms of nearly three-quarters of a century—ending the era of Siena's greatest stability and prosperity.

ABRAHAM L. UDOVITCH (b. 1933), professor of
Near Eastern studies at Princeton University, focuses
his research upon the economic and social history of
the medieval Islamic world. He is the author of
Partnership and Profit in Medieval Islam (1970). In
the following selection he takes issue with accepted
scholarly views and posits a new thesis concerning the
role of the Black Death in the history of Muslim
Egypt.*

Abraham L. Udovitch

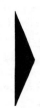

Egypt: Crisis in a Muslim Land

In very broad outline, the basic argument of what may be described as the current consensus explaining Egypt's economic decline runs as follows: The political unrest preceding and following the accession of the Circassian Mamlūks[1] in 1382 resulted in internal turmoil and weakness. The loosening of state control encouraged increased bedouin encroachments on agricultural areas and on caravans resulting in the decline of rural goods production, the flight of the rural population, the loss of cultivated lands to the desert and a disruption of lucrative long-distance trade. The most disastrous consequence of internal Mamlūk dissension was the adverse effect on agricultural revenues which were their fundamental source of wealth. Diminishing agricultural revenues were in turn the ultimate source of urban economic problems, since these directly affected the level of income of the urban upper classes and exerted pressure for a variety of economically disruptive measures such as heavier taxation of urban commerce, confiscations,

[1] The Mamluks were regiments of slaves who overthrew the Egyptian government in 1250 and established one of their number as sultan. They replenished their ranks during the thirteenth and fourteenth centuries by purchasing more slaves, for example, from Genoese merchants.—Ed.

*Abraham L. Udovitch, "Egypt," pt. IV of Robert Lopez, Harry Miskimin, Abraham L. Udovitch, "England to Egypt, 1350–1500: Long-term Trends and Long-distance Trade," from *Studies in the Economic History of the Middle East* edited by M. A. Cook (1970) and published by Oxford University Press for the School of Oriental and African Studies, pp. 117–120. Most footnotes omitted.

and forced purchases, all intended to buttress sagging Mamlūk incomes. This led to a descending spiral of urban economic decay to which our data on industrial and commercial decline bear such eloquent testimony.

I submit that this analysis is an inadequate explanation both of the extent and the manifestations of Egypt's economic crisis. A number of questions are left unanswered. Since bedouin disruption of agriculture began as early as the 1330's, why are there no indications of any disastrous long-term consequences until much later in the fourteenth century? Similarly, oppressive exactions from both the urban and agricultural sectors were not novel features of Mamlūk rule. Why, then, in earlier periods, did these not lead to any pervasive and calamitous economic decline? The most important question left unanswered is: how did Egypt continue to feed itself in the face of diminishing agricultural production? If the area of land under cultivation and the absolute size of the agricultural harvest declined by a considerable percentage, and if the population remained relatively constant, we would expect a number of consequences to follow: either mass starvation, or a sustained inflation in the price of agricultural products, or both. Since we have no evidence that either of these occurred, nor of any continuing massive grain imports, we must conclude that demographic factors were at the root of Egypt's agricultural decline, and that smaller harvests were being produced by, and were feeding substantially fewer people.

While a number of scholars have posited a slow but steady demographic decline in Egypt beginning with the Islamic conquest and continuing to the time of Muhammad 'Alī in the early nineteenth

century, this process was certainly accelerated in the mid-fourteenth century, becoming a significant, and indeed, a central factor in the history of the following century. The only population studies of this period are found in Ayalon's investigations of the Mamlūk army.[2] These reveal a drastic reduction in the number of Mamlūks beginning in the late fourteenth or early fifteenth century. From an estimated 12,000 royal Mamlūks during the reign of Nāṣir Muḥammad (first half of the fourteenth century), their number fell to approximately 5,500 under Mu'ayyad Shaykh in 1417, and to about 4,000 in 1437 under Barsbāy. Other segments of the Mamlūk army suffered a similar decline in numbers, so that "most of the military expeditions concerning which Egyptian chronicles of the fifteenth century give details were carried out by two or three thousand, and sometimes, by several hundred Mamlūks." Whatever political and other factors contributed to the precipitate reduction in the size of the Mamlūk army, the decimations of the plague were undoubtedly the most important. The plague took a particularly heavy toll in Mamlūk ranks, since as imported foreigners their immunity was low and they were particularly vulnerable; it also decreased the population source in the Caucasus on which the Manlūks drew for their manpower needs.

The plague did not confine its devastations only to the Mamlūks. All strata of the Egyptian population suffered from the destructive impact of the series of plagues which visited Egypt during the latter half of the fourteenth and throughout the fifteenth centuries. Any recovery from the demographic inroads of these

[2] D. Ayalon, "Studies on the Structure of Mamluk Army I," *Bulletin of the School of Oriental and African Studies*, XV (1953), 222–228.

epidemics was made virtually impossible by their recurrence at intervals of between ten and twenty years. Maqrīzi[3] has left us a vivid description of the progress of what was probably the most costly outbreak of the plague, that of 1347–9. It made its appearance in Egypt in the autumn of 1347. By April 1348 it had spread throughout the country, attaining its height between November 1348 and January 1349, and finally subsiding in February 1349. During this year and a half it wreaked its havoc throughout Egypt from Alexandria in the North to the outskirts of Aswān in the South. In Alexandria, the plague carried off one hundred people each day, and at its height this number rose to two hundred. The royal tirāz[4] factory was closed down for lack of workers; the markets and custom houses suspended operations for lack of merchants and travellers. The Delta areas were similarly afflicted. "In Maḥalla the plague was so intense that the prefect (wālī) could find no one to come to complain to him; and the qāḍī,[5] when approached by people to validate their wills, could, because of their small number, find no witnesses except after great exertion." In the countryside, there was almost no one left to cultivate the land or collect the harvests. Fief-holders and their servants were forced to gather the harvest themselves. Even though they held out one-half of the harvest as a reward to anyone who would help, they could find no one to accept their offer. Because of the heavy toll taken from the army, fiefs rapidly passed from one person to another, changing hands as many as seven or

eight times. Even artisans such as tailors and cobblers were falling heir to fiefs; and these latter mounted horses and donned military dress. Following the visitation of the plague, an expanse of land in Upper Egypt which was previously inhabited by 6,000 taxpayers contained only 116 who could pay taxes. In Cairo the number of daily deaths rose from 300 at the beginning of October 1348 to 3,000 towards the end of the month. Many streets were left only with empty houses, "and the belongings of their occupants could not find a taker; and if a man inherited anything, it passed in one day to a fourth and a fifth party." Survivors helped themselves to abandoned property, houses, furniture and money. Maqrīzi claims that in Cairo alone 900,000 people died, and that the figure would be doubled were it to include some of its suburbs and adjacent areas.

While Maqrīzi's figures for Cairo are certainly exaggerated, his description is unequivocal in portraying the plague as a serious demographic blow to all parts of Egypt. At this stage of research, it is impossible to give any quantitative or comparative figures for the extent of the population decline. One can only say with certainty that it was considerable. In another of his works, Maqrīzi reports that in this period the Egyptian population declined by one-third. In view of almost identical European figures this would seem to be a reasonable estimate and, until more detailed and controlled studies are available, one which can be used for a working hypothesis.

Postulating a serious demographic decline in the mid-fourteenth century permits us to view the consequent economic decline in a new perspective. The causal relationship explaining the crisis can now be reversed. It was not rapacious Mamlūk policies which led to decline, it

---

[3] The historian Maqrīzi (d. 1442) wrote a valuable and voluminous history of early Mamlūk Egypt. —Ed.

[4] Tirāz was embroidered cloth, ordinarily silk, intended for consumption by the royal court.—Ed.

[5] The qāḍī were judges whose purview included notarial matters.—Ed.

was rather the decline that was responsible for those policies. Demographic decline resulted in an absolute reduction of both urban and rural economic activity, thus accounting for a good deal, though not necessarily all, of the desolation described in our sources. Because of the uneven effects of the demographic decline on the price structures of the urban and rural sectors ... the Mamlūk ruling classes and the state generally, for whom agricultural revenues constituted the most important single source of income, were particularly hard hit. Higher urban prices and relatively lower agricultural profits impelled the government to squeeze the rural areas for more revenues and to intensify their taxation of, and expand their intervention into, urban commerce.

Suggested Additional Readings

A student of the Black Death might well begin with Philip Ziegler, *The Black Death* (New York and London, 1969), a very useful survey despite its author's modesty. Ziegler devotes far more space to the plague in England than elsewhere, and is weakest in dealing with the plague's agricultural and cultural effects. His imaginative reconstruction of "The Plague in a Medieval Village" (chap. 13) would be an excellent point of departure for the beginning student. The book contains one of the two most useful bibliographies on the plague, although it is marred by several errors and peculiarities of citation that make its use needlessly difficult.

Essential to any study of the plague is Élisabeth Carpentier, "Autour de la peste noire: famines et épidémies dans l'histoire du XIVe siècle," *Annales. Économies, Sociétés, Civilisations,* XVII (1962), 1062–1092. This extended bibliographic essay surveys most of the important recent literature and summarizes scholarly debates on the subject. The use of Ziegler and Carpentier will lead the student to much of the important literature concerning the Black Death.

It would be fatuous to offer here the bibliographies of Ziegler and Carpentier. Rather, I will suggest some studies that have appeared since they were published or that they omit, and a few of the more interesting older works.

The general survey by George Deaux, *The Black Death, 1347* (London, 1969) is superficial, chatty, and rambling. Its principal offering consists of snippets from chronicles, letters, etc., related to the plague in European history; but the lack of scholarly apparatus makes it extremely difficult for a reader to find the printed editions of those sources. More convenient for one wishing to dip into translated source materials is Johannes Nohl, *The Black Death. A Chronicle of the Plague,* translated by C. H. Clarke (London, 1926), of which an abridged paperback version is available (London: Unwin Books, 1961). A much briefer and less pretentious survey, though confined to the mid-fourteenth-century plague (and not entirely satisfactory) is a good student paper by Tony Godfrey-Smith, "Plague and the Decline of Medieval Europe: Correlation or Coincidence?" in *Australian National University Historical Journal,* I (1964), 13–43. Far more valuable is the wide-ranging article by Édouard Perroy, "À l'origine d'une économie contractée: les crises du XIVe siècle," *Annales. Économies, Sociétés, Civilisations,* IV (1949), 167–182, which holds that crises of 1315–1320 in agriculture, 1335–1345 in finance and money, and 1348–1350 in demography had a "paralyzing action on the economy" and kept it contracted for a century.

For an introduction to the medical aspects of the plague, see Leonard Fabian Hirst, *The Conquest of Plague. A Study of the Evolution of Epidemiology* (London, 1953) and R. Pollitzer, *Plague* (Geneva, 1954).

Michael M. Postan has produced and stimulated much valuable scholarship. In "Some Evidence of Declining Population in the Later Middle Ages," *Economic History Review,* ser. II, vol. II (1950), 221–246, he sets forth in greater detail the views so briefly summarized in his article in this book, and relates them to the claims of earlier scholarship. See also his "The Fifteenth Century," *Economic History Review,* IX (1939), 160–167. His position was challenged directly by W. C. Robinson, "Money, Population and Economic Change in Late Medieval Europe," *Economic History Review,* ser. II, vol. XII (1959), 63–76; to which Postan replied on pp. 77–82 of the same issue. Well worth reading is Barbara F. Harvey, "The Population Trend in England between 1300 and 1348," *Transactions of the Royal Historical Society,* ser. V, vol. XVI (1966), 23–42. She contends that "As from the movement of rents, so from the topography of settlement, we might conclude that the population trend was fairly stable in the first half of the fourteenth century.... Perhaps ... we do not need to add this half-century to the periods of history when the death-rate and not the birth-rate has exercised the more profound influence on the population trend."

The question of preplague population calls to mind the stimulating studies of Josiah Cox Russell. One might proceed from his *British Medieval Population* (Albuquerque, N.M., 1948) to *Late Ancient and Medieval Population,* Transactions of the American Philosophical Society, n.s., vol. XLVIII, pt. 3 (Philadelphia, 1958); and then to such articles as "Late Mediaeval Population Patterns," *Speculum,* XX (1945), 157–171; "Demographic Pattern in History," *Population Studies,* I (1947–1948), 388–404; "A Quantitative Approach to Medieval Population Change," *Journal of Economic History,* XXIV (1964), 1–21; "Recent Advances in Mediaeval Demography," *Speculum,* XL (1965), 84–101; or the more specialized "The Medieval Monedatge of Aragon and Valencia," *Proceedings of the American Philosophical Society,* CVI (1962), 483–504. *Comparative Studies in Society and History,* VIII (1966) contains Russell's valuable "Effects of Pestilence and Plague, 1315–1385," pp. 464–473, and a comment upon it by Sylvia Thrupp, pp. 474–479.

Before considering the Black Death in relation to specific regions we might note another small part of the growing literature concerning the economic trends of the late Middle Ages and the Renaissance and the role of the plague. Here a key figure is Robert S. Lopez. See especially Robert S. Lopez and Harry A. Miskimin, "The Economic Depression of the Renaissance," *Economic History Review,* ser. II, vol. XIV (1962), 408–426; and the debate among Lopez, Miskimin, and Carlo M. Cipolla, "Economic Depression of the Renaissance?" *Economic History Review,* ser, II, vol. XVI (1964), 519–529, in which Cipolla challenges the position of Lopez and Miskimin. (These articles might be read in conjunction with the selection in this book from Kosminskii.)

A large literature deals with the plague in various lands and nations. For England, one should now consult J. F. D. Shrewsbury, *A History of the Bubonic Plague in the British Isles* (London, 1970). This book by an emeritus professor of bacteriology at the University of Birmingham treats the period from the Middle Ages through the seventeenth century and has a useful bibliography. Still to be read is John Saltmarsh, "Plague and Economic Decline in England in the Later Middle Ages," *Cambridge Historical Journal,* VII (1941), 23–41; and the counter by J. M. W. Bean, "Plague, Population and Economic Decline in England in the Later Middle Ages," *Economic History Review,* ser. II, vol. XV (1963), 423–437, which contends that endemic plague did not lead to continuous population decline in the fourteenth and fifteenth centuries. See also Johan Schreiner, "Wages and Prices in England in the Later Middle Ages," *Scandinavian Economic History Review,* II (1954), 61–73. For those concerned with Scandinavia who do not read the languages of that region, it is fortunate that Schreiner's *Pest og prisfall in senmiddelalderen* (Oslo, 1948) contains an English summary (pp. 120–123).

The notes in the articles by Delatouche, Henneman, and Perroy will lead one to a considerable literature on the plague in France. See especially Yves Renouard, "Conséquences et intérêt démographiques de la peste noire de 1348," *Population,* III (1948), 459–466, and Philippe Wolff, "Trois études de démographie mediévale en France méridionale," *Studi in onore di Armando Sapori,* I (Milan, 1957), 493–503, which summarizes the work of three of Wolff's students. Wolff concludes that contemporaries had a right to be horrified, as perhaps as much as half of the population died in the mid-fourteenth-century epidemic; but that we must "not exaggerate the social consequences of the disaster. It does not seem to have overturned the social system." See also Richard W. Emery, "The Black Death of 1348 in Peripignan," *Speculum*, XLII (1967), 611–623. Those who do not read French might still derive some profit from Helen Robbins, "A Comparison of the Effects of the Black Death on the Economic Organization of France and England," *Journal of Political Economy*, XXXVI (1928), 447–479.

Essential to a consideration of the plague in Germany are Wilhelm Abel, *Die Wüstungen des ausgehenden Mittelalters*, 2d ed. (Stuttgart, 1955); Friederick Lütge, "Das 14./15. Jahrhundert in der Sozial- und Wirtschaftsgeschichte, *Jahrbücher für Nationalöknomie und Statistik*, CLXII (1950), 161–213; and Ernst Kelter, "Das deutsche Wirtschaftsleben des 14. und 15. Jahrhunderts im Schatten der Pestepidemien," in the same periodical, CLXV (1953), 161–208. Kelter sees crises in Germany much like those discussed by Lütge; but while Lütge places a great part of the blame on the plague of 1348, Kelter would stress the role of *recurrent* outbreaks of the epidemic coupled with fear of famine.

There is no comprehensive study of the plague for Spain or Italy analogous, for example, to that of Shrewsbury for the British Isles; hence some quite old studies still have certain value. See, for example, Alfonso Corradi, *Annali delle epidemie occorse in Italia dalle prime memorie fino al 1850*, 8 vols. (Bologna, 1865–1894); Maxim Kovalevsky, *Die ökonomische Entwicklung Europas bis zum Beginn der kapitalistischen Wirtschaftsformen*, V (Berlin, 1911), especially chaps. 6, 7 (re: Italy & Spain), pp. 277–321, 321–362. For Spain, see particularly the studies of A. Lopez de Meneses, such as, "Documentos acerca de la peste negra en los dominios de la corona de Aragón," *Estudios de Edad media*

de la Corona de Aragón. Sección de Zaragoza de la Escuela de estudios medievales del Consejo superior de investigaciones cientificas, VI (Saragossa, 1956), 291–447. For insights into the impact of the Black Death upon Russian history, see Gustave Alef, "The Crisis of the Muscovite Aristocracy: A Factor in the Growth of Monarchical Power," *Forschungen zur osteuropäischen Geschichte*, XV (1970), 16–68.

Closely related topics should be considered in connection with any broad study of the Black Death. Particularly fascinating is J. C. Russell, "That Earlier Plague," *Demography*, V (1968), 174–184, which deals with the great sixth-century epidemic. In it Russell suggests that "The plague interrupted and probably made impossible" the Emperor Justinian's program "of reestablishing the whole Roman Empire. . . ." For the controversial famines of the early fourteenth century one might turn first to Henry S. Lucas, "The Great European Famine of 1315, 1316 and 1317," *Speculum*, V (1930), 343–377. The extensive bibliography (pp. 835–845) appended to Léopold Genicot's most useful "Crisis: From the Middle Ages to Modern Times," the concluding chapter (VIII, pp. 660–741) in *The Cambridge Economic History of Europe*, vol. I, 2d ed. (London, 1966), cites a wealth of literature on such themes as "Demographic Trends and their Factors" and "Prices and Wages" as well as some items (pp. 840–841) that deal specifically with the plague. Students would do well to read the issue of *Annales. Économies, Sociétés, Civilisations*, XXIV, no. 6 (November–December, 1969), devoted entirely to "Histoire Biologique et Société;" and, in fact, *Annales. Économies, Sociétés, Civilisations* is the scholarly periodical most likely to keep one informed of the newest developments and approaches in the historiography of the Black Death.